Keto Vegan Air Fryer Cookbook

The Most Wanted and Irresistible Plant-Based Protein and Low-Carb Recipes to Air Fry, Roast, Bake, and Grill at Home

Written By

Linda Rea

Veggie wontons

INGREDIENTS

- 30 wonton wrappers
- 3/4 cup cabbage, grated
- 1/2 cup white onion, grated
- 1/2 cup carrot, grated
- 1/2 cup mushrooms, chopped
- 3/4 cup red pepper, chopped
- 1 tablespoon chili sauce
- 1 teaspoon garlic powder
- 1/2 teaspoon white pepper
- Pinch of salt
- 1/4 cup water
- Spray olive oil

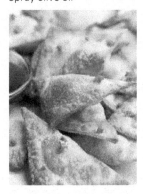

COOKING STEPS

1. Sauté cabbage, onion, carrot, mushrooms, and red pepper with olive oil in a skillet until soft.
2. Mix chili sauce, white pepper, salt, and garlic powder, then pour in the vegetables.
3. Stir and cook for 2 minutes until well mixed.
4. Remove the filling from the heat and allow it cool.
5. Spread the wonton wrappers on the working surface.
6. Add 1 tablespoon of vegetable filling on top of each wrapper.
7. Wet their edges, then fold each wrapper in half and roll them in a wonton.
8. Place the wrapped wontons in the air fryer basket.
9. Return the basket to the air fryer.
10. Select the air fry mode at 320 degrees f for 6 minutes. Serve warm.
11. You can serve with red chunky salsa or chili sauce.
12. Add ground chicken to the filling.

Nutrition: Calories 193 Fat 1g Carbs 37g Fiber 6g Sugar 9g Protein 6g

Copyright 2021 © [Linda Rea]

Legal & Disclaimer

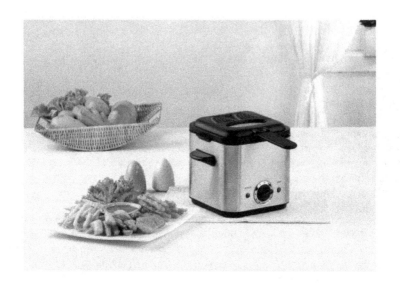

Keto Vegan (6) Air Fryer

TABLE OF CONTENS

Easy rosemary green beans 77

Sriracha golden cauliflower 78

Cauliflower tater tots 79

Chili fingerling potatoes 80

Golden pickles 81

Garlic eggplant slices 82

Lemony falafel 83

Crispy chickpeas 84

Spicy roasted potatoes 85

Skinny pumpkin chips 86

Mediterranean vegetable skewers 87

Fried peppers with sriracha mayo 88

Spinach with groundnuts 89

Chili roasted eggplant soba 90

Fettuccini with roasted vegetables in tomato sauce 91

Brown rice, spinach and tofu frittata 92

Coconut curry vegetable rice bowls 93

Tofu with Sticky Orange Sauce 94

Green beans and shallots 95

Toasty pepper bites 96

Platter of brussels and pine nuts 97

Vegetable Spring Rolls 98

Onion Pakora 99

Introduction

Veganism is fast catching up with many people across the world. The noble idea behind veganism, such as not wanting to exploit the less fortunate animal species of the world by taking what is theirs and selfishly using it for ourselves simply because they do not have the power to stop us, is perhaps, the primary reason for the growth in popularity of this concept.

However, in addition to the above extremely thoughtful reason, the health benefits and other great things about veganism are all sufficiently powerful causes for the expansion of the idea of veganism across the planet. This book is written with an intention to exhort newcomers to try a one-month vegan challenge that has the power to change not just your lifestyle but your entire outlook on life.

Before you decide to try to change your lifestyle to vegan, there are a few things you must know and understand about it. This book aims to do exactly that by giving you a detailed overview in the following areas:

- What is veganism?
- A brief history on veganism
- How is veganism useful to you?
- Meal plans for a one-month challenge along with recipe outlines
- How to stay committed to the cause?

WHAT IS VEGANISM?

You know who vegetarians are? They do not consume poultry, meat, or fish in their diet. Vegans, additionally, do not consume or use any animal products and/or by-products such as dairy products, honey, eggs, leather, silk, fur, and soaps and cosmetics made from animal sources. Vegans are the superset of vegetarians. All vegans are also vegetarians but all vegetarians need not be vegans.

Vegans believe that veganism is not just about their diet but a way of life. As far as possible, vegans avoid exploitation of animals in any form including but not limited to food, clothing, or other purposes. They also avoid items that have been tested on animals before being commercialized. And believe it or not, there is a vegan diet for all kinds of diets ranging from the junk food lovers to the raw food lovers and those in between, too.

HISTORY OF VEGANISM

Veganism, although not known as veganism, has been around for many centuries. Examples of prevention of exploitation against and cruelty to animals have been written in history books. Lord Buddha of India and Pythagoras both advocated this concept and had put in rules to ensure their followers ate only plant-based food and completely avoided meats and animal products.

The earliest modern-day veganism is known to have occurred around 1806 CE. During that time, the great English poet P. B. Shelley and Dr. William Lambe publicly objected to consuming dairy products and eggs by humans on ethical grounds. This incident seems to have laid the foundation for modern-day veganism.

In November 1944, six non-dairy vegetarians including Donald Watson and Elsie Shrigley met together and discussed the topic on non-dairy vegetarians' lifestyles and diets. Despite strong opposition, these six members founded the new movement and became actively involved in this new project.

This book deals only with the dietary aspect of veganism, giving you ample sufficient reasons to shift your lifestyle to this healthy and noble one. While the benefits of turning vegan are discussed in another chapter, the kind of foods that you can include in your diet while keeping your energy levels and health not just unchanged but also improved than earlier is huge.

Here is a small list of foods that are known to be totally vegan:

- **All kinds of grains and cereals**
- **All kinds of beans and legumes**
- **All fruits and vegetables**

Other vegan foods include soy milk, vegan mayonnaise, vegan ice cream and cheese, vegan hot dogs, and more. Moreover, a lot of companies have come out with mock meats that give vegans a sense of eating meat. This book also has four chapters dedicated to making vegan foods, which includes easy-to-make recipes.

Why Go Vegan?

Most people in the world want to do the following things by some means or the other:

- Lose weight
- Eat better
- Get fitter and healthier
- Do something for society and the world at large

The great news is that if you shift to a vegan diet, you can achieve all the above goals. And let me assure you, you will enjoy delicious, wholesome, and satiating meals as well.

No loss or reduction in energy levels – There is a misconception that changing to a vegan diet reduces your energy levels. There are numerous unworthy talks of vegans living only on water and a few greens and hence their energy levels have taken a huge dip. And on the other side of the spectrum, there are plenty of spurious rumors that say going vegan is helping them do impossible things. These other-end-of-the-spectrum talks make out vegans to be people who can walk on water! Let me assure you that neither of the extremes is true or based on any scientific studies.

Health benefits are huge when you choose to go vegan. Of course, the initial learning curve is going to be steep and you would have to counter multiple challenges. However, once you have overcome these tough phases and complete the 30-day challenge, you are going feel to happier, lighter, and fit. Moreover, there multiple studies done by various organizations including the British Dietetic Association that has proven the excellent efficacies of getting fitter and healthier by following a vegan diet.

Here is the list of a few magic foods that can restore energy instantaneously:

Bananas – Already beautifully and naturally packaged by nature, this wonderful tropical fruit is normally the first you must reach out for when you feel tired or fatigued.

Walnuts – Another great pick-me-up tree nut, walnuts are rich in plant proteins, omega fatty acids, and vitamins giving you the almost-instant energy boost.

Green smoothies – Delicious smoothies made by tossing together strawberries, bananas, and orange juices are great and extremely healthy pick-me-ups to fight fatigue.

Coconut water – This is nature's energy drink and is amazingly refreshing and is filled with vitamins and potassium.

Kiwi – This low-fat delicious fruit is an instant energy enhancer triggered by the simple sugars present in it.

Why I chose to mention vegan energy boosters in the beginning itself is to help you overcome doubts regarding your ability to get on with your daily schedule if you choose to go vegan. Today there are many sportspeople who have shifted to this diet to keep fitter and sustain energy levels. So, if highly active people in the field of sports can take advantage of veganism, it should not be difficult for moderately active people like us to take this 30-day challenge and come out with flying colors.

Other great reasons to take the one-month challenge to go vegan are:

Lose weight and yet remain energized – Many of us would love to find a sensible way to lose excess weight and yet remain healthy and fit. Average vegans are known to weigh 20 pounds lesser than average meat-eaters. Despite this, vegan diets do not starve you and make you feel enervated like the usual run-of-the-meal fad diets do.

Keep diseases and health disorders away – The Academy of Nutrition and Dietetics have conducted multiple studies which show that taking the vegan route helps you steer clear of common disorders such as diabetes, hypertension or high blood pressure thereby preventing the onset of many modern-day diseases such as heart attacks, kidney failure, and others.

Vegan foods are yummy and delicious – If you thought going vegan means you would have to give up your favorite ice creams, hamburgers, and chicken sandwiches, then you are wrong. With demand for vegan products soaring, many companies are coming up with amazingly delicious vegan options that taste very much like the non-vegetarian stuff. You will not miss any of the meats and animal products at all. There are plenty of established brands that cater to veganism and deliver really tasty dairy and meat substitutes.

Vegan diets are full of highly nutritious and healthy food items including whole grains, beans and legumes, nuts, soy products, and fresh fruits and vegetables. Here are some of the health benefits that these fiber-rich and healthy food sources provide you with:

- **Minimal saturated fats** – Meats and dairy products contain plenty of saturated fats thereby increasing the risk of cardiovascular diseases. Vegan diets automatically reduce intake of saturated fats enhancing your health condition
- **Fiber** – A vegan diet is high in fiber content that is very conducive to healthy bowel movements.
- **Magnesium** – Dark, green leafy vegetables are a rich source of magnesium, a key element that aids the body in the absorption of calcium.
- **Potassium** – Similarly, potassium, an important mineral that balances acidity and water in our body and helps in the removal of toxins, is found plenty in plant-based foods.
- **Proteins** – Meat-eaters invariably end up with more proteins than is needed by the body. Vegan diets, which include nuts, beans, and legumes, have the right amount of proteins for us.

Vegan diets provide other critically essential nutrients such as Vitamins E and C, phytochemicals, antioxidants, and foliate. These help in keeping your immunity system healthy and robust, and also prevent age-related diseases such as Alzheimer's and Parkinson's disease and keep your overall body organs functioning well.

Vegan diets have the power to prevent the following diseases that are very common in today's high-stress unhealthy lifestyle:

- Cardiovascular diseases
- Reduced cholesterol due to the complete absence of meat and dairy products in your diet
- Age-related macular degeneration
- Reduced risk of breast cancer
- Reduced risk of contracting ailments like diabetes, hypertension, cataracts, colon and prostate cancer, arthritis, and osteoporosis

In addition to improved health and prevention of diseases, going vegan makes you stronger, more energetic, and more attractive. Here is how:

Lowered Body Mass Index – Cutting meat and dairy out of your diet naturally reduces Body Mass Index.

Weight loss – Weight loss is an unquestioned effect of a vegan diet.

Healthy skin – Consuming rich sources of Vitamins A and E from nuts and fruits and vegetables enhance the texture and health of your skin.

Reduced allergy symptoms – Plant-based foods do not trigger as many allergic reactions in humans as dairy and meat products do

Less intake of mercury – A lot of shellfish and fish contain high levels of mercury, which we take in when we eat these foods. Switching to veganism does away with this toxin completely.

The above are only some of the great reasons that you must start off this 30-day vegan challenge. Instead of finding reasons not to do something good, focus on the above reasons which tell you why you should do it and dive straight in. Summon some extra willpower and after you complete this challenge you can rest assured that the willpower would come on its own when you see and feel the wondrous new VEGAN YOU.

What are the benefits an Air Fryer?

As you are aware, an air fryer is a great appliance to have in your kitchen. Not only does it save on the time taken to cook, but it also produces healthy meals. It's worthwhile looking at some of the health benefits provided by it.

- Healthy foods

The air fryer is quite popular, owing to producing healthy meals. It reduces oils and fats, thereby making the result relatively healthy. The same cannot be said about standard cooking techniques where you must add in lots of oils and fats. These can adversely affect your health and be the reason for obesity and illnesses. Therefore, an air fryer is best suited for improving their health by making changes in their cooking habits.

- Time

The time crunch is one of the most significant issues people face today and age, as everybody is preoccupied with one thing or another. The air fryer effectively solves this problem, as you can prepare foods within a short period. It works by cutting down on 20% of the time taken to cook foods the traditional way. This feature comes in handy for many people, including working professionals, students, and the elderly. If you are always short of time, then it is best to invest in an air fryer as soon as you get a chance.

- Usage

The air fryer is extremely easy to use and can be used by just about anyone. The machine is supplied with a manual that can be used to operate the appliance. The manual will also provide you with the right temperatures and times to cook different meals. With time, you will know the exact measures and be able to cook meals much faster. However, it will take a certain level of trial and error to stumble upon the right temperatures and times until you get used to using it. Remember, your ideas center around traditional cooking.

- Effort required

The air fryer is designed to be a very efficient machine that pretty much works by itself. It means that you don't have to put in too much effort to operate it. You just have to prepare the ingredients and add them to the appliance, and it will take it from there. You don't have to sauté, season, cover or keep an eye on the foods you place into the oven. All these steps are eliminated, thereby reducing both your effort and time taken to cook a meal. It makes it ideal for all those who are usually too lazy to cook up a meal and prefer takeout.

- Nutritional content

An air fryer helps maintain food's nutritional value. Cooking foods at higher temperatures can cause nutritional value to deplete. This issue is solved with an air fryer as it retains the nutritional content of foods placed into it.

- Cost of cooking

The air fryer helps in cutting down on the overall costs of cooking. It cuts down on the use of oils and fats, thereby reducing the overall costs of providing your family with food. Another advantage of cooking with an air fryer is that it tends to expand the food item, thereby decreasing the quantity required to cook a meal, reducing cooking costs. You will be surprised by the reduction in your budget and overall cooking costs.

- Variety in cooking

Throwing parties and cooking big meals will now be quite easy thanks to the air fryer's multitasking ability. One of the most advantages of using an air fryer is that it can be used for many different cooking purposes. Right from roasting to frying to baking, the air fryer can be put to many uses. You can also use it to grill foods, making it a truly versatile appliance to have in your kitchen. What's more, you will have the choice of cooking several dishes at the same time by using the separator provided with the fryer.

- Maintaining the fryer

It is easy to maintain the air fryer, as you do not have to do too much to stay clean. You can eliminate the need to clean several appliances and get away with cleaning, just one that servings many purposes. The machine is easy to clean from the outside. The basket and catching utensil are dishwasher friendly.

- Cost saving

The air fryer is quite cheap, price wise, considering the utility that it can provide. You don't need to buy different appliances like an oven, a grill, a chip fryer, etc. It can be done through the air fryer alone. Think of it as a onetime investment that is sure to last you a lifetime if taken care of following manufacturer instructions. Always read these, as the maintenance of each fryer will differ.

These descriptions show the different benefits of using air fryer. Each one of these contributes towards making it an ideal appliance to have in your kitchen.

ANY TIPS ON USING AIR FRYER?

An air fryer is a little device that has rapidly grown in popularity in the last few years. It is supposed to help you bake food. Some people call them air fryer ovens. You may remember when you saw your first Indian dish inspired by food fried in oil. Now, it's time to take you on a tour of the world and in a healthier way!

In the last few years, air fryers have become more and more popular. A lot of websites and blogs are now making them out to be the new microwave oven or rice cooker. The fine folks at Amana, pioneers in air fryers, sent me one of their most hot selling models.

Frying has become a bad word lately. As a result, we try to cut down on it in as many of our recipes as possible. Fortunately, air fryers are a great way to make food taste like it's been fried when it hasn't. So, here are some tips on cooking with air fryers:

Air fryers are available in multiple sizes. Look for one that fits the amount of food you want to make. Some air fryers are small enough that you would only use them for a snack or a single person. Others could make enough food for a whole family. There's also a market for commercial sized air fryers, and they're quite large. They could make enough food for a dozen people easily. They're also versatile in that they can be used for baking and as steamers.

Your new air fryer comes with a lot of accessories. You don't need to worry too much about them at the moment. Here are a few tips.

1. No matter what your air fryer comes with, you'll also need a pan and a spatula. The pan is for use as a defroster and a catch-all for when you take out the food. The spatula is to get food out of the air fryer. Remember that the food comes out very hot, so use caution.

2. Look at the shape of your air fryer. It may be a square or a circle. You can do a lot of things to a square air fryer, but few to a circle one. Look at your recipe and decide what you want to use it for.

3. The air fryer's controls are arguably the most important part. The air fryer has a lot of temperature controls that are quite precise. Unlike a microwave oven, an air fryer can give you a wide range of temperatures. You can cook things at really low temperatures, and you can cook things at incredibly hot temperatures that you couldn't use otherwise. Of course, you can also use it at the default temperature. Use the recommendations for your model in the instruction manual to help figure out which temperature is best for your needs.

4. You can make very unique recipes using the air fryer. The temperature and the food you use set the tone of the meal. The temperature you want to use should depend mostly on the type of food you're making, or even how you want it to come out. Low temperature cooking is helpful when you want to cook things slowly. You also want foods with a lot of moisture to be cooked at a high temperature because they cook through faster. You can make dishes with vegetables and meats evenly. You can also make quick breads since they would take less time and the other ingredients are easier to get.

5. Air fryers are very inexpensive. No matter what your budget is, there is an air fryer that fits it. They're mainly used for snacks. However, you can use the air fryer for other recipes if you want. They're a great alternative to the waffle iron, and you can cook a wide range of foods with them.

6. There are different components to an air fryer, and you can use each of them for different purposes. The top is traditionally used for eggs and for

steaming. The middle can be used for both frying foods and steaming them. The bottom is typically for fries and other fried foods.

7. Air fryers are very versatile. It's hard to find a recipe that can't be used in an air fryer. It's possible to make chicken legs, wings, and even drumsticks. You can even make foods with breading. People can even make grills and pizzas in air fryers.

8. If you're looking for the best air fryer, you can't go wrong with a Norpro. This is a great air fryer that is affordable and very easy to use. It has multiple functions and will work in no time.

9. Most air fryers have a filter. You need to make sure you always keep the filter cleaned. As much as you don't want to clean your air fryer, you have to clean the filter. This is very important because all the cooking oil is retained in the filter.

10. There are different types of air fryers. The ones that are made of glass and stainless steel are the most expensive. They're also more attractive. There are the ones that are made of plastic. Finally, there are the ones that are made from non-stick surfaces. These are the cheapest and also the most commonly sold air fryers.

Now you have in your hands all the information needed to safely proceed toward your Mediterranean lifelong transformation to increase your Health, your Confidence and your Vitality. Using your Air Fryer will also guarantee you delicious and time effective recipes that will help you integrate the foundational Habits of Health into your everyday routine. By incorporating the Habits of Health into your new lifestyle, you will be able to take your first steps towards the life you wish for. You will feel restored, more confident and your energy levels will be up. Enjoy life to the fullest.

Eating Healthy

If you haven't already been tracking your "macros and micros" for your regular vegan diet, it's about time that you started. There is no better way to make sure you're getting the exact amount of calories, and the exact amount of nutrients, that your body needs without tracking your macros and micros. "Macros" is an abbreviation that stands for "macronutrients," and they're what the Keto diet is based on. The three main macronutrients required for human life are carbohydrates, proteins, and fats. That's right! Tracking your macronutrients is just as easy as tracking how many grams of protein, carbohydrates, and fats you're eating in each meal. It does get a bit more complicated than that, but it's nothing you won't be able to handle. "Micros," then, stands for "micronutrients," and these are quite different from what you might be thinking. Micronutrients are actually the vitamins and minerals that your body requires to function, and micros are often essential for macros to do their jobs. Without the help of certain minerals, our macronutrients wouldn't be able to synthesize new proteins, add in our cellular regeneration, and help move bad molecules like harmful cholesterol out of our arteries. In order to make sure you're getting your proper dosages of micronutrients, you take supplements! One of the many helpful connections between veganism and the Keto diet is that both tend to require a healthy amount of added vitamins and minerals. Check back to **Chapter 1** if you need a refresher. However, it's worth noting that there are many more suggested micronutrients that we're supposed to get per day beyond just the popular five or seven. In fact, there are a whopping twenty-five micronutrients that our diets are supposed to provide us with every day. Although some of the amounts are so small, they're measured in micrograms—it's worth taking a look at this list to know what else you might want to supplement.

A multivitamin in combination with your regular vegan diet supplements should supply you with the perfect amount of each of these smaller micronutrients. You should, however, consult your physician before you start taking iron supplements. Tracking your macronutrients is definitely more involved, but there's a special tool that we're going to borrow from the body-building community to make it easier.

How Weighing Your Portions Ensures Success:

Nobody likes a scale, but isn't it true that everything's better when there's food involved? Back when the fitness community began to really focus on how our diets were facilitating weight loss, many body-builders and intense athletes started to use food scales as a way to be more precise about the portion sizes. But not just portions of whole meals—weighing your food with a food scale allows you to calculate the number of macronutrients **and** the number of calories in each portion of the meals you're going to prepare each week. The first step to using your food scale is to download an app called MyFitnessPal (the most popular macronutrient tracking app out there, and a great community to get involved with if you're vegan!). If you don't have a smartphone, feel free to use an online calculator—you'll be able to find more than a few. The next step is to visit your local restaurant supply store to stock up on large containers. Each week, when you prepare your meal on Sunday, you'll want to use your food scale to weight the entire cooked meal (all three or four portions together). To do this, set your chosen container on your scale and make the numbers read "00.00" – you're going to be pouring your entire meal into these containers to measure, so bigger is better. Once you've measured the full meal, use your application to plug in each of the ingredients you used in the meal and their amounts. This is just another reason that it's important to be organized with your grocery shopping. The resulting numbers should give you the number of total calories and nutrients, and if you divide by the number of portions you intend for the meal to make, you'll have an accurate nutritional label of calories, vitamins, and nutrients.

PREPARE TO MEAL PREP:

Meal prep, short for meal preparation, is a technique known far and wide in the fitness community as one of the best ways to ensure that you're eating a protein-packed, well-balanced meal with the proper portions to maximize your weight loss (or gain) without taking up too much time. During the week, most of us work forty hours or more—and if you're adding in the time that it takes to go to the gym, commute back and forth, finish your weekly work, and manage whatever other responsibilities you have—there isn't much time left for home-cooking. However, the meals you might purchase at a supermarket or restaurant simply won't fit in with a strict diet, especially one that combines two strict methods of eating. Meal prep is a great technique for busy individuals to use to make sure that they're getting the proper amount of fats, proteins, and carbohydrates for their diet and fitness. When you're eating a vegan Keto diet, you want to pay extra attention to the breakdown of nutrients in your food (and how those nutrients measure up in terms of carbohydrate content). Skip down to the section titled "Meal Prep Tips for Vegans Eating Keto" to get a better handle on your nutrient breakdown if you're already familiar with how to meal prep. If you aren't, everything you need to know is right below.

HOW TO MEAL PREP:

The idea behind meal prepping is incredibly simple, but the timing is a little less self-explanatory. Meal prepping is a practice that takes place normally on a Sunday before the work week begins when most people have enough time to cook multiple large-batch meals in one day. Yes, you'll most likely end up cooking more meals on Sunday than you'll get to eat. It's alright. You'll thank yourself late in the week. Meal prepping on Sundays normally starts with a trip to the grocery store to make sure your produce is as fresh as possible. While some more advanced meal prep specialists have adapted to using their freezer for fresh ingredients, you'll only want to rely on your freezer for full meals at the beginning of your journey. Normally meal prep consists of all the dinner, lunches, breakfasts, and snacks you can possibly prepare to give yourself time to go to the gym and get enough sleep while you're working. The easiest way to tackle meal prep for the first time is to start by making four lunches and four dinners in one Sunday. Although that might seem like a fair amount, it's really only two meals that you'll be cooking in large batches. Meal prep is known for creating quite the large mess in the kitchen, so take the time to do a bit of pre-cleaning so that you won't regret it afterward. A pre-clean is a great time to make sure all your largest pots, saucepans, and skillets and ready to cook with; one meal might not always mean one pot. Many vegan Keto recipes rely on sautéing, steaming, and grilling in order to give a smoky depth of flavor to foods with a more neutral palette. While your gathering your cooking utensils, remember that meal prepping is all about organization. Before you go to the grocery store, make sure you have all your ingredients written down and that you know what to look for when it comes to labels. High carb content in both carbs and net carbs will impact your ability to reach Ketosis. Once you're ready to start cooking, make sure you have plenty of healthy cooking oils on hand to lubricate your pans. Coconut oil is recommended, but with its low smoke point, you're welcome to use olive oil if you need to cook hotter for longer. After you're finished, it's crucial that you have equal sized Tupperware for proper storage. Nothing ruins a good middle of the week meal like opening your squash spaghetti to freezer burn. Most cooked meals take three to five days to go bad, so while you don't have to put your prepped meals in the freezer, sometimes it's a good back up if your fridge is low on space. That's about all there is to the process of preparing your meals, but what about prepping meals specifically for a vegan Keto diet? Does anything change?

MEAL PREP TIPS FOR VEGANS EATING KETO

A vegan Keto diet isn't the most restrictive diet out there, but it's certainly one of the more admirable challenges in the health and fitness world. Sticking to a vegan Keto diet can be hard, but meal prepping the best vegan Keto meals will make a world of difference when it comes to upholding your commitment. Many of our lives are constantly busy, and when you're trying to maintain a Keto diet, it's imperative that you eat at the same time each day—especially if you're on a fast. This might mean eating at work or packing a meal to take with you for after the gym. Either way, preparing your necessary meals each week will give you more time to focus on your mental health and less time worrying about pounds that will melt off naturally. You'll also be able to portion out your carbs, fats, and proteins according to your Keto guidelines, which will help infinitely in organizing. As a vegan eating Keto, you'll also want to make sure that you're paying special attention to things like generated plastic waste—if you're trying to save the planet by eating less meat, it doesn't make much sense to package your snacks each day in disposable Ziploc baggies. Glass Tupperware are the cornerstones of vegan meal prep containers, and the many different sizes and tight lids of Mason jars are perfect for taking your snacks and salads on the go. But meal preparation is more than just saving you time, money, and precious calories. Portioning out your meals is a key part of both veganism and the Keto diet because of your need to more urgently check certain nutrition boxes. These nutrition boxes are called you macronutrients and micronutrients, and if fats, carbs, and proteins thought they were the only reason we portioned out or meals, they were very wrong. Tracking your "macros and micros" is just like making sure you don't eat too much bread in one day—except for your body, it's a lot more serious. These essential chemicals can sometimes mean the difference between a perfectly healthy body, and one that struggles to function.

.

Cooking Tips for Beans, Legumes, and Grains

1. Soak beans for at least 8 to 10 hours (preferably overnight) to remove any anti-nutrients. This reduces the chances of stomach cramps, gas, and bloating.

2. If you're pressed for time, you can also use a quick **Soak Method**. Just boil enough water to cover the beans, add in the beans, let simmer for 10 minutes, and set aside for an hour.

3. Soak quinoa and brown rice for a couple of hours. Lentils and other grains don't require any prior soaking.

COOKING UTENSILS

1. Cooking in a pressure cooker

Drain the water from one cup of previously soaked beans, grains, or lentils. Rinse the vegetables well and add them to a 6-to 8-quart cooker.

Add 2-4 cups of water. Close the lid and cook on high heat.

When the cooker reaches a high pressure, lower the heat, and cook for an extra 7-10 minutes. Turn off the heat, let everything cool, and open the lid.

2. Cooking in a slow cooker

Drain the water from one cup of previously soaked beans/quinoa/brown rice, rinse well, and add to a smaller slow cooker.

Pour in 2-4 cups of water. Add other ingredients except for salt (for stews, soups, and one pot meals). Cover the slow cooker with a lid and cook on high heat for 3-4 hours, or 7-8 hours on low heat. Add in salt in the last 10 minutes of cooking.

3. Cooking Grains and Lentils on a Stovetop

Respect the following quantities when cooking on a stove top. Water and Yield are measured in cups, and time in minutes.

WHY USING AN AIR FRYER FOR COOKING VEGAN DISHES?

If you already own (or you are thinking of buying) an **Air Fryer** you will have in your hands all the tools that will guarantee you top results. You can use your Air Fryer to cook all your vegan dishes from this cookbook in a quick and easy way, without compromising on taste and while staying within budget!

As you might already know, an air fryer is a small type of oven. It is an innovative countertop kitchen gadget that fries or cook's food by circulating hot air via convection current. The air fryer has a heating ring that produces hot air. There is also a mechanical fan that circulates the hot air all over the food at high speed. This hot air cook or fries the food to give the same crispy product as the oil fried variety. The difference between air frying and oil frying is that while oil frying involves immersion of the food into the hot oil to cook, the air fryer doesn't. It means that you can achieve the same cooking results as in oil frying but with little to no oil.

The air fryer works great for foods like roasted vegetables, especially roasted garlic, vegetables, grains, pulses and tofu. Most air fryers come with timers and temperature adjustments to make for more precise cooking. There is an opening at the top that takes in air, heated up by the heating rings, and subsequently blown over the food, thereby efficiently cooking them. A cooking basket also sits on top of a drip tray inside which the food is cooked. This basket needs to be shaken frequently to ensure even mixing of oil and a better cooking result. While most models have agitators that initiate this shaking at regular intervals, most others do not, and the shaking should be done manually.

Since air fryers don't require as much oil as oil frying does, they are generally considered healthier. An air fryer reduces the oil content of food to nearly

80% less than oil frying. It is because the food does not absorb as much oil as with oil frying. However, this difference has led to arguments about the taste of air fried food compared to the oil fried variety. Since oil adds more flavor to fried food as it is being absorbed, it comes as no surprise if an air fried food tastes slightly different from oil fried ones. An excellent example is French fries that may taste a lot different when air fried than the usual oil fried delicacy. Tofu, however, turns out pretty great whether sprinkled with oil or not before air frying.

Moreover, spraying the food with oil before air frying gives it an added crispiness compared to the one that was not sprinkled before air frying. Oil on its own is also one of the essential macronutrients and will come in handy in the right proportion.

There are many heart friendly oils out there, which you can spread over your food before air frying to achieve that fabulous taste. These oils can be used to sprinkle your food before air frying to maintain a healthier diet. Just like most innovative appliances, the air fryer might come with an initial dread on how to use it effectively. Once mastered, the art of air frying is what many people find themselves resorting to more often than not. Even though air frying is a convenient hands-off cooking method, using the air fryer is more than just turning on the device and leaving your kitchen.

- BREAKFAST

- BRUNCH

- LUNCH

- DINNER

- DESSERT

- FRUIT

- VEGETABLES

Breakfast banana oatmeal

5 minutes

12 minutes

Breakfast

04 Servings

INGREDIENTS

- 1 cup old-fashioned oats
- 1 cup of coconut milk
- 1 cup of water
- 1 banana, mashed
- 1/2 teaspoon vanilla extract
- 1/2 teaspoon ground cinnamon
- A pinch of grated nutmeg
- A pinch of sea salt

COOKING STEPS

1. Thoroughly combine all ingredients in a mixing bowl. Spoon the mixture into lightly greased mugs.
2. Then, place the mugs in the air fryer cooking basket.
3. Bake your oatmeal at 380 degrees f for about 12 minutes.

Nutrition: Calories 217 Fat 7g Carbs 34g Protein 8g

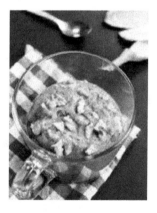

Old-fashioned granola

5 minutes

15 minutes

Breakfast

6 Servings

INGREDIENTS

- 1/2 cup rolled oats
- 1/4 cup wheat germ, toasted
- 1/2 cup dried cranberries
- 1/4 cup pumpkin seeds
- 1/4 cup sunflower seeds
- 1/4 cup pecans, chopped
- 1/4 cup walnuts, chopped
- 1/2 teaspoon vanilla extract
- 1/4 cup agave syrup
- 4 tablespoons coconut oil
- 1 teaspoon pumpkin pie

COOKING STEPS

1. Start by preheating your air fryer to 350 degrees f.
2. Thoroughly combine all ingredients in a lightly greased baking pan.
3. Then, place the pan in the air fryer cooking basket. Bake your granola for about 15 minutes, stirring every 5 minutes.
4. Stock in a closed container for up to three weeks.

Nutrition: Calories: 332 Fat: 19g Carbs: 38g Protein: 7g

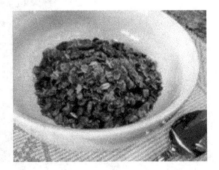

Mushroom and rice bake

5 minutes

10 minutes

Breakfast

4 Servings

INGREDIENTS

- 1pound brown mushrooms, chopped
- 1 small onion, peeled and chopped
- 2 tablespoons butter, room temperature
- 2 garlic cloves, minced
- Ground black pepper
- Sea salt, to taste
- 1 cup vegetable broth
- 1 ½ cups brown rice, cooked

COOKING STEPS

1. Put your air fryer to 360 degrees f.

2. Thoroughly combine all ingredients in a lightly greased baking pan.

3. Lower the pan into the air fryer cooking basket.

4. Cook for about 10 minutes or until cooked through.

Nutrition: **Calories: 192 Fat: 28g Carbs: 6g Protein: 3g**

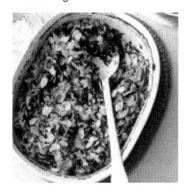

Cheesy cauliflower risotto

5 minutes   10 minutes   Breakfast   4 Servings

INGREDIENTS

Preparation time: 5 minutes

Cooking time: 10 minutes

Servings: 4

Ingredients:

- 2 cups rice, cooked
- 2 tablespoons olive oil
- 1/2 cup cauliflower, chopped
- 1/2 cup vegetable broth
- 4 tablespoons mozzarella cheese, shredded

COOKING STEPS

1. Prepare your air fryer to 360 degrees f.

2. Thoroughly combine all ingredients in a lightly greased baking pan.

3. Lower the pan into the air fryer cooking basket.

4. Cook for about 10 minutes or until cooked through.

Nutrition: Calories: 218 Fat: 11g Carbs: 25g Protein: 5g Sugars: 2g Fiber: 2g

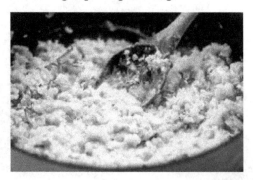

Autumn walnut porridge

10 minutes

15 minutes

Dessert

06 Servings

INGREDIENTS

Preparation time: 5 minutes

Cooking time: 10 minutes

Servings: 4

Ingredients:

- 1/2 cup rolled oats
- 1/2 cup rye flakes
- 1 cup milk
- 1 cup applesauce, unsweetened
- 1/2 cup walnuts, chopped
- A pinch of coarse sea salt
- A pinch of freshly grated nutmeg

COOKING STEPS

1. Thoroughly combine all ingredients in a mixing bowl.

2. Spoon the mixture into a lightly greased casserole dish.

3. Lower the dish into the air fryer cooking basket.

4. Bake your oatmeal at 380 degrees f for about 12 minutes.

Nutrition: Calories: 249 Fat: 10g Carbs: 33g Protein: 3g Sugars: 9g Fiber: 5g

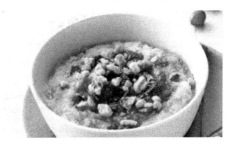

Morning potatoes

 10 minutes
 18 minutes
 Breakfast
 4 Servings

INGREDIENTS

- 2 medium russet potatoes, diced
- 1/2 teaspoon salt
- 1 tablespoon olive oil
- 1/4 teaspoon garlic powder
- Chopped parsley for garnish

COOKING STEPS

1. Dice the washed potatoes into half inch cubes.
2. Soak the potatoes in ice-cold water for 45 minutes.
3. Drain the potatoes and pat them dry.
4. Toss the potatoes with salt, garlic powder, and olive oil in a large bowl.
5. Set air fryer on fries mode for 18 minutes at 400 degrees f, then press preheat.
6. Once preheated, place the prepared potatoes in the basket, return it to the fryer, and press start.
7. Shake the potatoes when cooked halfway through, then resume cooking.
8. Garnish with parsley, then enjoy.

Nutrition: Calories 134 Fat7 g Carbohydrates 51 g Fiber 7 g Sugar 3 g Protein 2 g

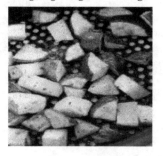

Kale potato nuggets

 15 minutes 18 minutes Breakfast 4 Servings

INGREDIENTS

- 2 cups potatoes, chopped
- 1 teaspoon olive oil
- 1 garlic clove, minced
- 4 cups kale, chopped
- 1/8 cup almond milk
- 1/4 teaspoon sea salt
- 1/8 teaspoon ground black pepper
- Vegetable oil spray as needed

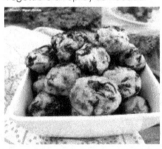

COOKING STEPS

1. Set a cooking pot filled with water over medium heat.
2. Add potatoes to this boiling water and cook for 30 minutes until soft.
3. Meanwhile, sauté garlic with oil in a skillet over medium high heat until golden.
4. Stir in kale and sauté for 3 minutes., then transfer this mixture to a bowl.
5. Drain the boiled potatoes and add them to the kale.
6. Mix the potatoes with a potato masher.
7. Stir in salt, black pepper, and milk them, mix well.
8. Make 1inch potato nuggets out of this mixture.
9. Place these nuggets in the air fryer basket.
10. Return the air fryer basket to the air fryer.
11. Select the air fry mode at 390 degrees f for 15 minutes.
12. Flip the nuggets once cooked halfway through, then resume cooking. Serve warm.

Nutrition: Calories 113 Fat 3g Carbs 20g Fiber 3g Sugar 1g Protein 5g

Air fried falafel

15 minutes   10 minutes   Breakfast   6 Servings

INGREDIENTS

- 1 1/2 cups dry garbanzo beans
- 1/2 cup fresh parsley, chopped
- 1/2 cup fresh cilantro, chopped
- 1/2 cup white onion, chopped
- 7 garlic cloves, minced
- 2 tablespoons all-purpose flour
- 1/2 teaspoons sea salt
- 1 tablespoon ground cumin
- 1/8 teaspoons ground cardamom
- 1 teaspoon ground coriander
- 1/8 teaspoons cayenne pepper

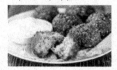

COOKING STEPS

1. Soak garbanzo beans in a bowl filled with water for 24 hours.
2. Drain and transfer the beans to a cooking pot filled with water.
3. Cook the beans for 1 hour or more on simmer until soft.
4. Add cilantro, onion, garlic, and parsley to a food processor and blend until finely chopped.
5. Drain the cooked garbanzo beans and transfer them to the food processor.
6. Add salt, cardamom, cayenne, coriander, cumin, and flour.
7. Blend until it makes a rough dough.
8. Transfer this falafel mixture to a bowl, cover with a plastic wrap and refrigerate for 2 hours.
9. Make 1 ½ inches balls out of this bean's mixture.
10. Lightly press the balls and place them in the air fryer basket.
11. Return the air fryer basket to the air fryer.
12. Select the air fry mode at 400 degrees f for 10 minutes.
13. Flip the falafels once cooked halfway through the resume cooking.
14. Serve warm.

Nutrition: Calories 206 Fat 4g Carbs 35g Fiber 4g Sugar 9g Protein 16g

Veggie bites

INGREDIENTS

- 1 large broccoli, cut into florets
- 6 large carrots, diced
- A handful of garden peas
- 1/2 cauliflower, riced
- 1 large onion, peeled and diced
- 1 small zucchini, diced
- 2 leeks, sliced
- 1 can coconut milk
- 2 oz. Plain flour
- 1 cm cube ginger peeled and grated
- 1 tablespoon garlic puree
- 1 tablespoon olive oil
- 1 tablespoon Thai green curry paste
- 1 tablespoon coriander
- 1 tablespoon mixed spice
- 1 teaspoon cumin
- Salt and black pepper, to taste

COOKING STEPS

1. Place leek and courgette in a steamer basket and steam them for 20 minutes.
2. Sauté onion, ginger, and garlic with olive oil in a skillet until soft.
3. Add steamed leek and courgette to the skillet and sauté for 5 minutes.
4. Stir in coconut milk and the rest of the spices.
5. Mix well, then add the cauliflower rice then cook for 10 minutes.
6. Remove the hot skillet from the heat and allow it to cool.
7. Cover and refrigerate this mixture for 1 hour.
8. Slice the mixture into bitesize pieces and place these pieces in the air fryer basket.
9. Return the air fryer basket to the air fryer.
10. Select the air fry mode at 350 degrees f for 10 minutes.
11. Carefully flip the bites once cooked halfway through, then resume cooking. Serve warm.

Nutrition: Calories 270 Fat 16g Carbs 33g Fiber 5g Sugar 7g Protein 4g

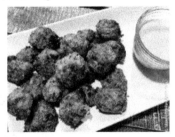

Fried mushrooms

 15 minutes   25 minutes   Breakfast   6 Servings

INGREDIENTS

Preparation time: 15 minutes

Cooking time: 25 minutes

Serving: 6

Ingredients:

- 2 cups oyster mushrooms
- 1 cup buttermilk
- 1 ½ cups all-purpose flour
- 1 teaspoon salt
- 1 teaspoon black pepper
- 1 teaspoon garlic powder
- 1 teaspoon onion powder
- 1 teaspoon smoked paprika
- 1 teaspoon cumin
- 1 tablespoon oil

COOKING STEPS

1. At 375 degrees f, preheat your air fryer on air fry mode.
2. Clean the mushrooms and then soak them in buttermilk for 15 minutes.
3. Mix all-purpose flour with onion powder, garlic powder, black pepper, salt, smoked paprika, and cumin in a suitable bowl.
4. Coat the mushrooms with flour mixture and then dip again with buttermilk.
5. Coat the mushrooms again with flour and buttermilk.
6. Place the coated mushrooms in the air fryer basket.
7. Return the air fryer basket to the air fryer and cook for 10 minutes.
8. Flip the mushrooms once cooked halfway through. Serve warm.

Nutrition: Calories 166 Fat 2g Carbs 28g Fiber 8g Sugar 7g Protein 8g

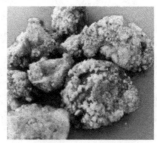

Parmesan eggplant

INGREDIENTS

Preparation time: 15 minutes

Cooking time: 15 minutes

Serving: 4

Ingredients:

- 1/2 cup flour
- 1/2 cup almond milk
- 1/2 cup panko breadcrumbs
- 2 tablespoons parmesan, grated
- Onion powder to taste
- Garlic powder to taste
- 1 large eggplant, stems removed and sliced
- Salt and black pepper, to taste
- Eggplant parmesan:
- 1 cup marinara sauce
- 1/2 cup mozzarella shreds
- Parmesan, grated

COOKING STEPS

1. Mix panko crumbs with garlic powder, black pepper, salt, onion powder, and vegan parmesan in a bowl.
2. First coat the eggplant slices with flour, then dip in the almond milk and finally coat with breadcrumbs mixture.
3. Place the coated eggplant slices in the air fryer basket.
4. Put the basket back to the air fryer.
5. Select the air fry mode at 390 degrees f for 15 minutes.
6. Flip the eggplant slices once cooked halfway through.
7. Place the eggplant slices on the serving plate and top them with marinara sauce and cheese. Serve warm.

Nutrition: Calories 231 Fat 9g Carbs 38g Fiber 4g Sugar 7g Protein 3g

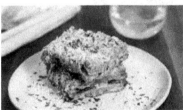

Black bean burger

INGREDIENTS

- 1 1/3 cups rolled oats
- 16 ounces canned black bean
- 3/4 cup salsa
- 1 tablespoon soy sauce
- 1 1/4 teaspoon mild chili powder
- 1/41/2 teaspoon chipotle chile powder
- 1/2 teaspoon garlic powder
- 1/2 cup corn kernels

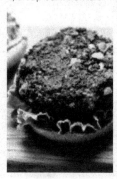

COOKING STEPS

1. Add all the rolled oats to a food processor and pulse to get a coarse meal.
2. Add black beans, salsa, soy sauce, chili powder, chile powder, and garlic powder.
3. .blend again for 1 minute, then transfer to a bowl.
4. Stir in corn kernel, then make six patties out of this mixture.
5. Place the black bean patties in the air fryer basket.
6. Return the air fryer basket to the air fryer.
7. Select the air fry mode at 375 degrees f for 15 minutes.
8. Flip the patties once cooked halfway through and resumed cooking.
9. Serve warm.

Nutrition: Calories 350 Fat 6g Carbs 66g Fiber 14g Sugar 3g Protein 19g

Potato cakes

INGREDIENTS

Preparation time: 10 minutes

Cooking time: 35 minutes

Serving: 4

Ingredients:

- 4 cups potatoes, diced
- 1 bunch green onions, chopped
- 1 lime, zest, and juice
- 1 1/2 inch knob of fresh ginger
- 1 tablespoon tamari
- 4 tablespoons red curry paste
- 4 sheets nori, chopped
- 1 can heart of palm, drained
- 3/4 cup canned artichoke hearts, drained
- Black pepper, to taste
- Salt, to taste

COOKING STEPS

1. Add potato cubes to a pot filled with water.
2. Place it over medium heat and cook until potatoes are soft.
3. Clear the potatoes and transfer them to a suitable bowl.
4. Mash the potatoes with a masher, then add green onions, lime juice, and remaining ingredients.
5. Mix well and stir in artichoke shreds.
6. Stir well and make 4 patties out of this mixture.
7. Place the patties in the air fryer basket.
8. Return the basket to the air fryer.
9. Select the air fry mode at 375 degrees f for 10 minutes.
10. Flip the patties once cooked halfway through and resume cooking. Serve warm.

Nutrition: Calories 208 Fat 5g Carbs 31g Fiber 8g Sugar 5g Protein 9g

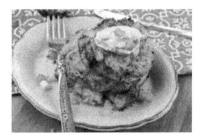

Veggie wontons

15 minutes   8 minutes   Breakfast   15 Servings

INGREDIENTS

- 30 wonton wrappers
- 3/4 cup cabbage, grated
- 1/2 cup white onion, grated
- 1/2 cup carrot, grated
- 1/2 cup mushrooms, chopped
- 3/4 cup red pepper, chopped
- 1 tablespoon chili sauce
- 1 teaspoon garlic powder
- 1/2 teaspoon white pepper
- Pinch of salt
- 1/4 cup water
- Spray olive oil

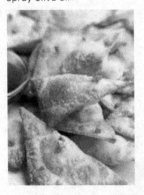

COOKING STEPS

13. Sauté cabbage, onion, carrot, mushrooms, and red pepper with olive oil in a skillet until soft.
14. Mix chili sauce, white pepper, salt, and garlic powder, then pour in the vegetables.
15. Stir and cook for 2 minutes until well mixed.
16. Remove the filling from the heat and allow it cool.
17. Spread the wonton wrappers on the working surface.
18. Add 1 tablespoon of vegetable filling on top of each wrapper.
19. Wet their edges, then fold each wrapper in half and roll them in a wonton.
20. Place the wrapped wontons in the air fryer basket.
21. Return the basket to the air fryer.
22. Select the air fry mode at 320 degrees f for 6 minutes. Serve warm.
23. You can serve with red chunky salsa or chili sauce.
24. Add ground chicken to the filling.

Nutrition: Calories 193 Fat 1g Carbs 37g Fiber 6g Sugar 9g Protein 6g

Garlic mogo chips

20 minutes

25 minutes

Breakfast

4 Servings

INGREDIENTS

- Mogo chips
- 1 lb. Mogo chips
- Salt to taste
- 1/2 teaspoon turmeric powder
- 1/2 teaspoon garlic powder
- 1 tablespoon lime juice
- 1/2 teaspoon oil
- 8 cups of water
- Masala mix
- 1 teaspoon red chili powder
- Pinch dried chili flakes
- 1/2 teaspoon garlic powder
- Salt to taste
- 1 teaspoon lime juice
- 1/2 teaspoon lime zest
- 1 teaspoon oil

COOKING STEPS

1. Mix water with oil, lime juice, turmeric powder, garlic powder, and salt in a saucepan.
2. Stir In mogo chips and cook for 8-10 minutes until the chips are boiled.
3. Drain and allow the chips to cool.
4. Mix all the spices for masala mix in a suitable bowl.
5. Toss in mogo chips and mix well to coat.
6. Spread the chips in the air fryer basket.
7. Return the air fryer basket to the air fryer.
8. Select the air fry mode at 400 degrees f for 5 minutes.
9. Toss the chips once cooked halfway through, then resume cooking. Serve warm.

Nutrition: Calories 212 Fat 18g Carbs 26g Fiber 4g Sugar 8g Protein 3g

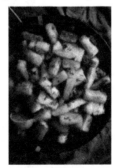

Simple and easy croutons

10 minutes   15 minutes   Dessert   06 Servings

INGREDIENTS

Preparation time: 5 minutes

Cooking time: 8 minutes

Servings: 4

Ingredients:

- 2 slices friendly bread
- 1 tablespoon olive oil

Hot soup, for serving

COOKING STEPS

1. Cut the slices of bread into medium-sized chunks.
2. Brush the air fryer basket with the oil and place the chunks inside.
3. Select the air fry function and cook at 390ºf (199ºcfor 8 minutes.
4. Serve with hot soup.

Nutrition: Calories: 120 Fat: 9g Carbs: 10g Protein: 2g Sugars: 2g Fiber: 0g

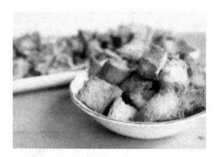

Cheesy potato patties

15 minutes   10 minutes   Breakfast   8 Servings

INGREDIENTS

- 2 pounds (907 g) white potatoes
- 1/2 cup finely chopped scallions
- 1/2 teaspoon ground black pepper
- 1 tablespoon fine sea salt
- 1/2 teaspoon hot paprika
- 2 cups shredded colby cheese
- 1/1 cup canola oil
- 1 cup crushed crackers

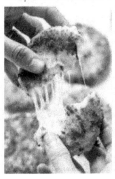

COOKING STEPS

1. Select the bake function and preheat to 360ºf (182ºc).
2. Boil the potatoes until soft. Dry them off and peel them before mashing thoroughly, leaving no lumps.
3. Combine the mashed potatoes with scallions, pepper, salt, paprika, and cheese.
4. Mold the mixture into balls with your hands and press with your palm to flatten them into patties.
5. In a shallow dish, combine the canola oil and crushed crackers. Coat the patties in the crumb mixture.
6. Bake the patties for about 10 minutes, in multiple batches if necessary. Serve hot.

Nutrition: Calories: 245 Fat: 15g Carbs: 22g Protein: 7g Sugars: 5g Fiber: 2g

Bistro potato wedges

 10 minutes   13 minutes   Breakfast   4 Servings

INGREDIENTS

- 1pound (454 g fingerling potatoes, cut into wedges)
- 1 teaspoon extra virgin olive oil
- 1/2 teaspoon garlic powder
- Salt and pepper, to taste
- 1/2 cup raw cashews, soaked in water overnight
- 1/2 teaspoon ground turmeric
- 1/2 teaspoon paprika
- 1 tablespoon nutritional yeast
- 1 teaspoon fresh lemon juice
- 2 tablespoons to ¼ cup water

COOKING STEPS

1. Get a bowl and put the potato wedges, olive oil, garlic powder, and salt and pepper, making sure to coat the potatoes well.
2. Move potatoes to the air fryer basket. Select the air fry function and cook at 400ºf (204ºc for 10 minutes).
3. In the meantime, prepare the cheese sauce. Pulse the cashews, turmeric, paprika, nutritional yeast, lemon juice, and water together in a food processor. You can put more water to achieve your desired consistency.
4. When the potatoes are finished cooking, transfer to a bowl and add the cheese sauce on top. Air fry for an additional 3 minutes.
5. Serve hot.

Nutrition: Calories: 100 Fat: 5g Carbs: 18g Protein: 2g Sugars: 1g Fiber: 2g

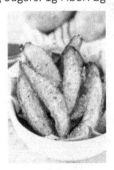

Breakfast Spinach Quiche

10 minutes

13 minutes

Breakfast

4 Servings

INGREDIENTS

- 7 ounces whole wheat flour
- 7ounces spinach, torn
- 2 tablespoons olive oil
- 2 tablespoons flax meal mixed with 3 tablespoons water
- 2 tablespoons almond milk
- 3 ounces soft tofu, crumbled
- Salt and black pepper to the taste
- 1 yellow onion, chopped

COOKING STEPS

1. In your food processor, mix flour with half of the oil, flax meal, milk, salt and pepper and pulse well.
2. Transfer to a bowl, knead a bit, cover and keep in the fridge for 10 minutes.
3. Heat up a pan with the rest of the oil over medium-high heat, add onion, spinach, tofu, salt and pepper, stir, cook for a few minutes and take off heat.
4. Divide dough in 4 pieces, roll each piece, place on the bottom of a ramekin, divide spinach mix into the ramekins, place all ramekins in your air fryer's basket and cook at 360 degrees F for 15 minutes.
5. Leave quiche aside to cool down a bit and then serve them for breakfast.
6. Enjoy!

Nutrition: calories 250, fat 12, fiber 2, carbs 13, protein 9

Greek Veggie Mix

10 minutes　　13 minutes　　Breakfast　　4 Servings

COOKING STEPS

Preparation time: 10 minutes

Cooking time: 45 minutes

Servings: 4

Ingredients:

- 8 ounces eggplant, sliced
- 8 ounces zucchini, sliced
- 8 ounces bell peppers, chopped
- 2 garlic cloves, minced
- 5 tablespoons olive oil
- 1 bay leaf
- 1 thyme spring
- 2 onions, chopped
- 8 ounces tomatoes, cut into quarters
- Salt and black pepper to the taste

1. Heat up a pan that fits your air fryer with 2 tablespoons oil over medium-high heat, add eggplant, salt and pepper, stir, cook for 5 minutes and transfer to a bowl.
2. Heat up the pan with 1 more tablespoon oil, add zucchini, cook for 3 minutes and transfer over eggplant pieces.
3. Heat up the pan again, add bell peppers, stir, cook for 2 minutes and pour over the other veggies.
4. Heat up the pan with 2 tablespoons oil, add onions, stir and cook for 3 minutes.
5. Add tomatoes, the rest of the veggies, bay leaf, thyme, garlic, salt and pepper, stir, transfer to your air fryer and cook at 300 degrees F for 30 minutes.
6. Divide between plates and serve for breakfast.
7. Enjoy!

Nutrition: calories 200, fat 1, fiber 3, carbs 7, protein 6

Tofu Casserole

10 minutes   20 minutes   Breakfast   4 Servings

INGREDIENTS

Preparation time: 10 minutes

Cooking time: 20 minutes

Servings: 4

Ingredients:

- 1 teaspoon lemon zest, grated
- 14 ounces tofu, cubed
- 1 tablespoon lemon juice
- 2 tablespoons nutritional yeast
- 1 tablespoon apple cider vinegar
- 1 tablespoon olive oil
- 2 garlic cloves, minced
- 10 ounces spinach, torn
- ½ cup yellow onion, chopped
- ½ teaspoon basil, dried
- 8 ounces mushrooms, sliced
- Salt and black pepper to the taste
- ¼ teaspoon red pepper flakes
- Cooking spray

COOKING STEPS

1. Spray your air fryer with some cooking spray, arrange tofu cubes on the bottom, add lemon zest, lemon juice, yeast, vinegar, olive oil, garlic, spinach, onion, basil, mushrooms, salt, pepper and pepper flakes, toss, cover and cook at 365 degrees F for 20 minutes.
2. Divide between plates and serve for breakfast.
3. Enjoy!

Nutrition: calories 246, fat 6, fiber 8, carbs 12, protein 4

Simple Granola

10 minutes   15 minutes   Breakfast   3 Servings

INGREDIENTS

- ½ cup granola
- ½ cup bran flakes
- 2 green apples, cored, peeled and roughly chopped
- ¼ cup apple juice
- 1/8 cup maple syrup
- 2 tablespoons cashew butter
- 1 teaspoon cinnamon powder
- ½ teaspoon nutmeg, ground

COOKING STEPS

1. In your air fryer, mix granola with bran flakes, apples, apple juice, maple syrup, cashew butter, cinnamon and nutmeg, toss, cover and cook at 365 degrees F for 15 minutes
2. Divide into bowls and serve for breakfast.
3. Enjoy!

Nutrition: calories 188, fat 6, fiber 9, carbs 11, protein 6

Greek Veggie with Thyme

10 minutes   45 minutes   Breakfast   4 Servings

INGREDIENTS

- 8 ounces eggplant, sliced
- 8 ounces zucchini, sliced
- 8 ounces bell peppers, chopped
- 2 garlic cloves, minced
- 5 tablespoons olive oil
- 1 bay leaf
- 1 thyme spring
- 2 onions, chopped
- 8 ounces tomatoes, cut into quarters
- Salt and black pepper to the taste

COOKING STEPS

1. Heat up a pan that fits your air fryer with 2 tablespoons oil over medium-high heat, add eggplant, salt and pepper, stir, cook for 5 minutes and transfer to a bowl.
2. Heat up the pan with 1 more tablespoon oil, add zucchini, cook for 3 minutes and transfer over eggplant pieces.
3. Heat up the pan again, add bell peppers, stir, cook for 2 minutes and pour over the other veggies.
4. Heat up the pan with 2 tablespoons oil, add onions, stir and cook for 3 minutes.
5. Add tomatoes, the rest of the veggies, bay leaf, thyme, garlic, salt and pepper, stir, transfer to your air fryer and cook at 300 degrees F for 30 minutes.
6. Divide between plates and serve for breakfast.
7. Enjoy!

Nutrition: calories 200, fat 1, fiber 3, carbs 7, protein 6

Tomatoes Breakfast Salad

10 minutes   20 minutes   Breakfast   2 Servings

INGREDIENTS

- 2 tomatoes, halved
- Cooking spray
- Salt and black pepper to the taste
- 1 teaspoon parsley, chopped
- 1 teaspoon basil, chopped
- 1 teaspoon oregano, chopped
- 1 teaspoon rosemary, chopped
- 1 cucumber, chopped
- 1 green onion, chopped

COOKING STEPS

1. Spray tomato halves with cooking oil, season with salt and pepper, place them in your air fryer's basket and cook at 320 degrees F for 20 minutes.
2. Transfer tomatoes to a bowl, add parsley, basil, oregano, rosemary, cucumber and onion, toss and serve for breakfast.
3. Enjoy!

Nutrition: calories 100, fat 1, fiber 3, carbs 8, protein 1

Veggie Casserole with Cashew

10 minutes

16 minutes

Breakfast

4 Servings

INGREDIENTS

Preparation time: 10 minutes

Cooking time: 16 minutes

Servings: 4

Ingredients:

- 2 teaspoons onion powder
- ¾ cup cashews, soaked for 30 minutes and drained
- ¼ cup nutritional yeast
- 1 teaspoon garlic powder
- ½ teaspoon sage, dried
- Salt and black pepper to the taste
- 1 yellow onion, chopped
- 2 tablespoons parsley, chopped
- 3 garlic cloves, minced
- 1 tablespoon olive oil
- 4 red potatoes, cubed
- ½ teaspoon red pepper flakes

COOKING STEPS

1. In your blender, mix cashews with onion powder, garlic powder, nutritional yeast, sage, salt and pepper and pulse really well.
2. Add oil to your air fryer's pan and preheat the machine to 370 degrees F.
3. Arrange potatoes, pepper flakes, garlic, onion, salt, pepper and parsley in the pan,
4. Add cashews sauce, toss, cover and cook for 16 minutes
5. Divide between plates and serve for breakfast.
6. Enjoy!

Nutrition: calories 218, fat 6, fiber 6, carbs 14, protein 5

Easy Breakfast Oats

 10 minutes   15 minutes   Breakfast   4 Servings

INGREDIENTS

- 2 cups almond milk
- 1 cup steel cut oats
- 2 cups water
- 1/3 cup cherries, dried
- 2 tablespoons cocoa powder
- ¼ cup stevia
- ½ teaspoon almond extract
- For the sauce:
- 2 tablespoons water
- 1 and ½ cups cherries
- ¼ teaspoon almond extract

COOKING STEPS

1. In your air fryer's pan, mix almond milk with oats, water, dried cherries, cocoa powder, stevia and ½ teaspoon almond extract, stir, cover and cook at 360 degrees F for 15 minutes.
2. Meanwhile, in a small pot, mix 2 tablespoons water with 1 and ½ cups cherries and ¼ teaspoon almond extract, stir, bring to a simmer over medium heat and cook for 10 minutes.
3. Divide oats into bowls, drizzle cherry sauce all over and serve for breakfast.
4. Enjoy!

Nutrition: calories 172, fat 7, fiber 7, carbs 12, protein 6

Lemony Tofu Casserole

10 minutes   20 minutes   Breakfast   4 Servings

INGREDIENTS

- 1 teaspoon lemon zest, grated
- 14 ounces tofu, cubed
- 1 tablespoon lemon juice
- 2 tablespoons nutritional yeast
- 1 tablespoon apple cider vinegar
- 1 tablespoon olive oil
- 2 garlic cloves, minced
- 10 ounces spinach, torn
- ½ cup yellow onion, chopped
- ½ teaspoon basil, dried
- 8 ounces mushrooms, sliced
- Salt and black pepper to the taste
- ¼ teaspoon red pepper flakes
- Cooking spray

COOKING STEPS

1. Spray your air fryer with some cooking spray, arrange tofu cubes on the bottom, add lemon zest, lemon juice, yeast, vinegar, olive oil, garlic, spinach, onion, basil, mushrooms, salt, pepper and pepper flakes, toss, cover and cook at 365 degrees F for 20 minutes.
2. Divide between plates and serve for breakfast.
3. Enjoy!

Nutrition: calories 246, fat 6, fiber 8, carbs 12, protein 4

Bell Pepper and Beans Oatmeal

10 minutes

15 minutes

Breakfast

2 Servings

INGREDIENTS

Preparation time: 10 minutes

Cooking time: 15 minutes

Servings: 2

Ingredients:

- 1 cup steel cut oats
- 2 tablespoons canned kidney beans, drained
- 2 red bell peppers, chopped
- 4 tablespoons coconut cream
- A pinch of sweet paprika
- Salt and black pepper to the taste
- ¼ teaspoon cumin, ground

COOKING STEPS

1. Heat up your air fryer at 360 degrees F, add oats, beans, bell peppers, coconut cream, paprika, salt, pepper and cumin, stir, cover and cook for 16 minutes.
2. Divide into bowls and serve for breakfast.
3. Enjoy!

Nutrition: calories 173, fat 4, fiber 6, carbs 12, protein 4

Banana and Walnuts Oats

10 minutes

15 minutes

Breakfast

4 Servings

INGREDIENTS

- 1 banana, peeled and mashed
- 1 cup steel cut oats
- 2 cups almond milk
- 2 cups water
- ¼ cup walnuts, chopped
- 2 tablespoons flaxseed meal
- 2 teaspoons cinnamon powder
- 1 teaspoon vanilla extract
- ½ teaspoon nutmeg, ground

COOKING STEPS

1. In your air fryer mix oats with almond milk, water, walnuts, flaxseed meal, cinnamon, vanilla and nutmeg, stir, cover and cook at 360 degrees F for 15 minutes.
2. Divide into bowls and serve for breakfast.
3. Enjoy!

Nutrition: calories 181, fat 7, fiber 6, carbs 12, protein 11

Spicy cauliflower rice

10 minutes

22 minutes

Brunch

2 Servings

INGREDIENTS

- 1 cauliflower head, cut into florets
- 1/2 tsp cumin
- 1/2 tsp chili powder
- 6 onion spring, chopped
- 2 jalapenos, chopped
- 4 tbsp olive oil
- 1 zucchini, trimmed and cut into cubes
- 1/2 tsp paprika
- 1/2 tsp garlic powder
- 1/2 tsp cayenne pepper
- 1/2 tsp pepper
- 1/2 tsp salt

COOKING STEPS

1. Preheat the air fryer to 370 f.
2. Prepare food processor and put the cauliflower florets. Process until it looks like rice.
3. Transfer cauliflower rice into the air fryer baking pan and drizzle with half oil.
4. Place pan in the air fryer and cook for 12 minutes, stir halfway through.
5. Heat remaining oil in a small pan over medium heat.
6. Add zucchini and cook for 58 minutes.
7. Add onion and jalapenos and cook for 5 minutes.
8. Add spices and stir well. Set aside.
9. Add cauliflower rice to the zucchini mixture and stir well.
10. Serve and enjoy.

Nutrition: Calories 254 Fat 28 g Carbohydrates 13 g Sugar 5 g Protein 3 g

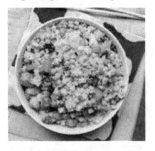

Radish hash browns

10 minutes

13 minutes

Brunch

4 Servings

INGREDIENTS

- 1 lb. Radishes, washed and cut off roots
- 1 tbsp olive oil
- 1/2 tsp paprika
- 1/2 tsp onion powder
- 1/2 tsp garlic powder
- 1 medium onion
- 1/4 tsp pepper
- 3/4 tsp sea salt

COOKING STEPS

1. Slice onion and radishes using a mandolin slicer.
2. Add sliced onion and radishes in a large mixing bowl and tossed with olive oil.
3. Transfer onion and radish slices to air fryer basket and cook at 360 f for 8 minutes. Shake basket twice.
4. Return onion and radish slices in a mixing bowl and toss with seasonings.
5. Again, cook onion, and radish slices in air fryer basket for 5 minutes at 400 f. Shake basket halfway through.
6. Serve and enjoy.

Nutrition: Calories 62 Fat 7 g Carbohydrates 1 g Sugar 5 g Protein 2 g

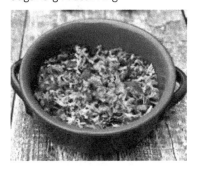

Air fried brussels sprouts

INGREDIENTS

- 1pound brussels sprouts
- 1 tablespoon coconut oil, melted

1 tablespoon unsalted butter, melted

COOKING STEPS

1. Preheat the air fryer oven to 400F (204C).
2. Prepare the Brussels sprouts by halving them, discarding any loose leaves.
3. Combine with the melted coconut oil and transfer to the air fryer basket. Set and cook for 10 minutes. Shake the basket once cooking. The sprouts are ready when they are partially caramelized.
4. Remove from the oven and serve with a topping of melted butter.

Nutrition: Calories: 45g Fat: 0g Carbs: 9g Protein: 2g

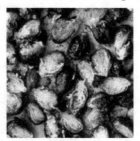

Easy rosemary green beans

5 minutes

5 minutes

Lunch

1 Servings

INGREDIENTS

- 1 tablespoon butter, melted
- 2 tablespoons rosemary
- 1/2 teaspoon salt
- 3 cloves garlic, minced
- 3/4 cup chopped green beans

COOKING STEPS

1. Preheat the air fryer oven to 390F (199C).
2. Combine the melted butter with the rosemary, salt, and minced garlic.
3. Toss in the green beans, coating them well. Transfer to the air fryer basket. Set air fryer time to 5 minutes.
4. Serve immediately.

Nutrition: Calories: 32 Fat: 3g Carbs: 8g Protein: 2g

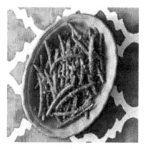

Sriracha golden cauliflower

15 minutes   17 minutes   Lunch   4 Servings

INGREDIENTS

- 1/4 cup vegan butter, melted
- 1/4 cup sriracha sauce
- 4 cups cauliflower florets
- 1 cup breadcrumbs
- 1 teaspoon salt

COOKING STEPS

1. Preheat the air fryer oven to 375F (191C).
2. Mix the sriracha and vegan butter in a bowl and pour this mixture over the cauliflower, taking care to cover each floret entirely.
3. Get another bowl. Mix the breadcrumbs and salt.
4. Dip the cauliflower florets in the breadcrumbs, coating each one well. Put them in the air fryer basket and set time to 17 minutes. Serve hot.

Nutrition: Calories: 469 Fat: 34g Carbs: 35g Protein: 15g

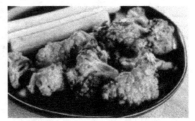

Cauliflower tater tots

INGREDIENTS

- 1pound (454 g) cauliflower, steamed and chopped
- ½ cup nutritional yeast
- 1 tablespoon oats
- 1 tablespoon desiccated coconuts
- 3 tablespoons flaxseed meal
- 3 tablespoons water
- 1 onion, chopped
- 1 teaspoon minced garlic
- 1 teaspoon chopped parsley
- 1 teaspoon chopped oregano
- 1 teaspoon chopped chives
- Salt and ground black pepper, to taste
- ½ cup breadcrumbs

COOKING STEPS

1. Preheat the air fryer oven to 375F (191C).
2. Drain any excess water out of the cauliflower by wringing it with a paper towel.
3. Mix the cauliflower with the remaining ingredients, save the breadcrumbs. Using the hands, shape the mixture into several small balls.
4. Coat the balls in the breadcrumbs and transfer to the air fryer
5. Change temperature to 400 degrees f and air fry for an additional 10 minutes.
6. Serve immediately.

Nutrition: Calories: 147 Fat: 6g Carbs: 20g Protein: 3g

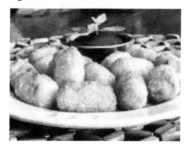

Chili fingerling potatoes

10 minutes

16 minutes

Lunch

4 Servings

INGREDIENTS

- 1pound (454 g) fingerling potatoes, rinsed and cut into wedges
- 1 teaspoon olive oil
- 1 teaspoon salt
- 1 teaspoon black pepper
- 1 teaspoon cayenne pepper
- 1 teaspoon nutritional yeast

  ½ teaspoon garlic powder

COOKING STEPS

1. Preheat the air fryer oven to 400F (204C).
2. Coat the potatoes with the rest of the ingredients. Transfer to the air fryer basket.
3. Place in the air fryer basket set time to 16 minutes, shaking the basket halfway through the cooking time.
4. Serve immediately.

Nutrition: Calories: 120 Fat: 4g Carbs: 20g Protein: 4g

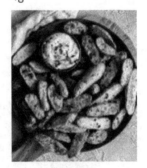

Golden pickles

10 minutes

15 minutes

Lunch

4 Servings

INGREDIENTS

- 14 dill pickles, sliced
- ¼ cup flour
- ⅛ teaspoon baking powder
- Pinch of salt
- 2 tablespoons cornstarch plus 3 tablespoons water
- 6 tablespoons panko breadcrumbs
- ½ teaspoon paprika
- Cooking spray

COOKING STEPS

1. Preheat the air fryer oven to 400F (204C).
2. Drain any excess moisture out of the dill pickles on a paper towel.
3. In a bowl, combine the flour, baking powder, and salt.
4. Throw in the cornstarch and water mixture and combine well with a whisk.
5. Put the panko breadcrumbs in a shallow dish along with the paprika. Mix thoroughly.
6. Dip the pickles in the flour batter before coating in the breadcrumbs. Spritz all the pickles with the cooking spray.
7. Transfer to the air fryer basket. Choose air fry and set time to 15 minutes, or until golden brown. Serve immediately.

Nutrition: Calories: 195 Fat: 13g Carbs: 20g Protein: 26g

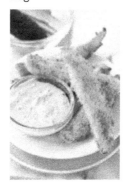

Garlic eggplant slices

5 minutes   15 minutes   Lunch   1 Servings

COOKING STEPS

Preparation time: 5 minutes

Cooking time: 15 minutes

Servings: 1

Ingredients:

- 1 large eggplant, sliced
- 2 tablespoons olive oil
- ¼ teaspoon salt
- ½ teaspoon garlic powder

1. Preheat the air fryer oven to 390F (199C).
2. Put eggplant slices with the olive oil, salt, and garlic powder in a mixing bowl until evenly coated.
3. Put the slices in the air fryer basket. Place the baking pan and cook for 15 minutes.
4. Serve immediately.

Nutrition: Calories: 66 Fat: 7g Carbs: 1g

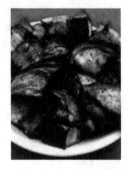

Lemony falafel

INGREDIENTS

Preparation time: 10 minutes

Cooking time: 15 minutes

Servings: 8

Ingredients:

- 1 teaspoon cumin seeds
- ½ teaspoon coriander seeds
- 2 cups chickpeas, drained and rinsed
- ½ teaspoon red pepper flakes
- 3 cloves garlic
- ¼ cup chopped parsley
- ¼ cup chopped coriander
- ½ onion, diced
- 1 tablespoon juice from freshly squeezed lemon
- 3 tablespoons flour
- ½ teaspoon salt
- Cooking spray

COOKING STEPS

1. Cook the cumin and coriander seeds over medium heat.
2. Grind using a mortar and pestle.
3. Put all ingredients, except for the cooking spray, in a food processor and blend until a fine consistency is achieved.
4. Use the hands to mold the mixture into falafels and spritz with the cooking spray.
5. Preheat the air fryer oven to 400F (204C).
6. Transfer the falafels to the air fryer basket in a single layer. Cook until golden brown. Serve warm.

Nutrition: Calories: 56 Fat: 1g Carbs: 9g Protein: 3g

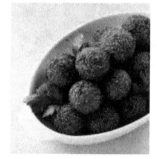

Crispy chickpeas

5 minutes

15 minutes

Lunch

4 Servings

INGREDIENTS

- 1 can (15ounces / 425gchickpeas, drained but not rinsed
- 2 tablespoons olive oil
- 1 teaspoon salt
- 2 tablespoons lemon juice

COOKING STEPS

1. Preheat the air fryer oven to 400ºf (204ºc).
2. Put and mix all ingredients in a bowl. Transfer this mixture to the air fryer basket.
3. Put mixture into baking pan and slide into rack position 2, select air fry, and set time to 15 minutes, ensuring the chickpeas become nice and crispy.
4. Serve immediately.

Nutrition: Calories: 132 Fat: 6g Carbs: 14g Protein: 5g

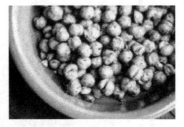

Spicy roasted potatoes

10 minutes · 12 minutes · Lunch · 2 Servings

COOKING STEPS

Preparation time: 10 minutes

Cooking time: 12 minutes

Servings: 2

Ingredients:

- 4 potatoes, peeled and cut into wedges
- 2 tablespoons olive oil
- Sea salt
- Ground black pepper, to taste
- 1 teaspoon cayenne pepper
- 1/2 teaspoon ancho chili powder

1. Get a bowl and mix all ingredients until the potatoes are well covered.
2. Transfer them to the air fryer basket and cook at 400 degrees f for 6 minutes. Shake the basket and cook for a further 6 minutes.
3. Serve warm with your favorite sauce for dipping. Enjoy!

Nutrition: Calories 299 Fat 16gCarbs 49g Protein 8g

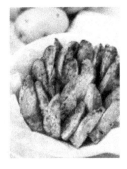

Skinny pumpkin chips

10 minutes   13 minutes   Lunch   2 Servings

INGREDIENTS

- 1pound pumpkin, cut into sticks
- 1 tablespoon coconut oil
- 1/2 teaspoon rosemary
- 1/2 teaspoon basil
- Salt and ground black pepper, to taste

COOKING STEPS

1. Start by preheating the air fryer to 395 degrees f. Brush the pumpkin sticks with coconut oil.
2. Put the spices and combine well.
3. Cook for 13 minutes, shaking the basket halfway through the cooking time.
4. Serve with mayonnaise. Bon appétit!

Calories 118 Fat 7g Carbs 17g Protein 2g

Nutrition: Calories 118 Fat 7g Carbs 17g Protein 2g

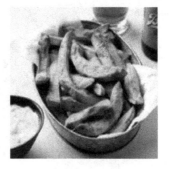

Mediterranean vegetable skewers

 15 minutes 13 minutes Lunch 4 Servings

INGREDIENTS

- 2 medium-sized zucchinis
- 2 red bell peppers
- 1 green bell pepper
- 1 red onion, cut into 1inch pieces
- 2 tablespoons olive oil
- Sea salt, to taste
- 1/2 teaspoon black pepper, preferably freshly cracked

  1/2 teaspoon red pepper flakes

COOKING STEPS

1. Cut the zucchinis, red and green bell peppers into 1inch pieces
2. Rinse the wooden skewers in water for 15 minutes.
3. Thread the vegetables on skewers; drizzle olive oil all over the vegetable skewers; sprinkle with spices.
4. Preheat at 400 degrees f and cook for 13 minutes. Serve warm and enjoy!

Nutrition: Calories 138Fat 12g Carbs 12g Protein 2g

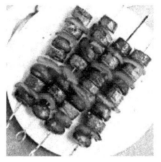

Fried peppers with sriracha mayo

10 minutes   14 minutes   Lunch   2 Servings

INGREDIENTS

Preparation time: 10 minutes

Cooking time: 14 minutes

Servings: 2

Ingredients:

- 4 bell peppers, seeded and sliced (1inch pieces
- 1 onion, sliced (1inch pieces)
- 1 tablespoon olive oil
- 1/2 teaspoon dried rosemary
- 1/2 teaspoon dried basil
- Kosher salt, to taste
- 1/4 teaspoon ground black pepper
- 1/3 cup mayonnaise
- 1/3 teaspoon sriracha

COOKING STEPS

1. Mix the onions and bell peppers with the olive oil, rosemary, basil, salt, and black pepper.
2. Place the peppers and onions on an even layer in the cooking basket.
3. Cook at 400 degrees f for 12 to 14 minutes.
4. Meanwhile, make the sauce by whisking the mayonnaise and sriracha. Serve immediately.

Nutrition: Calories: 15 Fiber: 5g Carbs: 5g Protein: 5g

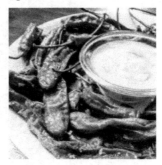

Spinach with groundnuts

10 minutes

15 minutes

Dinner

4 Servings

INGREDIENTS

- 1 tablespoon of ghee
- ½ tablespoon of red chili pepper
- ¼ tablespoon of cumin
- ½ teaspoon of salt
- ½ teaspoon of pepper
- 2 tomatoes
- 3 oz of groundnuts
- 6 oz of spinach
- 3 cloves of garlic
- ½ teaspoon of paprika
- ½ teaspoon of onion powder

COOKING STEPS

1. Wash and chop spinach in the pieces.
2. Then add red chili pepper, ghee, cumin, salt, pepper, groundnuts, garlic, paprika and onion powder.
3. Blend everything well.
4. After that chop tomatoes in the pieces.
5. Blend everything well.
6. Sprinkle the air fryer with oil.
7. Preheat it to 350f for 3 minutes.
8. Cook the meal in the air fryer for 10 minutes.
9. Then shake well and cook for 5 minutes more.
10. 1serve hot with parsley and basil leaves.

Nutrition: Calories: 103 Fat: 2,1g Carbohydrates: 3,8g Protein: 1,1g

Chili roasted eggplant soba

10 minutes

13 minutes

Dinner

4 Servings

INGREDIENTS

Basic recipe

Preparation time: 10 minutes

Cooking time: 15 minutes

Servings: 4

Ingredients:

- 200g eggplants
- Kosher salt
- Ground black pepper
- Noodles:
- 8 oz. Soba noodles
- 1 c. Sliced button mushrooms
- 2 tbsps. Peanut oil
- 2 tbsps. Light soy sauce
- 1 tablespoon rice vinegar
- 2 tbsps. Chopped cilantro
- 2 chopped red chili pepper
- 1 teaspoon sesame oil

COOKING STEPS

1. In a mixing bowl, mix together ingredients for the marinade.
2. Wash eggplants and then slice into ¼-inch thick cuts. Season with salt and pepper, to taste.
3. Preheat your air fryer to 390°f.
4. Place eggplants in the air fryer cooking basket. Cook for 10 minutes.
5. Meanwhile, cook the soba noodles according to packaging directions. Drain the noodles.
6. In a large mixing bowl, combine the peanut oil, soy sauce, rice vinegar, cilantro, chili, and sesame oil. Mix well.
7. Add the cooked soba noodles, mushrooms, and roasted eggplants; toss to coat.
8. Transfer mixture into the air fryer cooking basket. Cook for another 5 minutes.
9. Serve and enjoy!

Nutrition: calories 318 fat 2g carbs 54g protein 13g.

Fettuccini with roasted vegetables in tomato sauce

 10 minutes   25 minutes   Dinner   4 Servings

INGREDIENTS

- 10 oz. Spaghetti, cooked
- 1 eggplant, chopped
- 1 chopped bell pepper
- 1 zucchini, chopped
- 4 oz. Halved grape tomatoes
- 1 teaspoon minced garlic
- 4 tbsps. Divided olive oil
- Kosher salt
- Ground black pepper
- 12 oz. Can diced tomatoes
- ½ teaspoon dried basil
- ½ teaspoon dried oregano
- 1 teaspoon Spanish paprika
- 1 teaspoon brown sugar

COOKING STEPS

1. In a mixing bowl, combine together eggplant, red bell pepper, zucchini, grape tomatoes, garlic, and 2 tablespoons olive oil. Add some salt and pepper, to taste.
2. Preheat your air fryer to 390°f.
3. Place vegetable mixture in the air fryer cooking basket and cook for about 10-12 minutes, or until vegetables are tender. Meanwhile, you can start preparing the tomato sauce.
4. In a saucepan, heat remaining 2 tablespoons olive oil. Stir fry garlic for 2 minutes. Add diced tomatoes and simmer for 3 minutes.
5. Stir in basil, oregano, paprika, and brown sugar. Season with salt and pepper, to taste. Let it cook for another 5-7 minutes. Once cooked, transfer the vegetables from air fryer to a mixing bowl.
6. Add the cooked spaghetti and prepared a sauce. Toss to combine well.
7. Divide among 4 serving plates.
8. Serve and enjoy!

Nutrition: calories 330 fat 14g carbs 43g protein 9g.

Brown rice, spinach and tofu frittata

5 minutes

55 minutes

Dinner

4 Servings

INGREDIENTS

- ½ cup baby spinach, chopped
- ½ cup kale, chopped
- ½ onion, chopped
- ½ teaspoon turmeric
- 1 ¾ cups brown rice, cooked
- 1 flax egg (1 tablespoon flaxseed meal + 3 tablespoon cold water1 package firm tofu)
- 1 tablespoon olive oil
- 1 yellow pepper, chopped
- 2 tablespoons soy sauce
- 2 teaspoons arrowroot powder
- 2 teaspoons Dijon mustard
- 2/3 cup almond milk
- 3 big mushrooms, chopped
- 3 tablespoons nutritional yeast
- 4 cloves garlic, crushed
- 4 spring onions, chopped
- A handful of basil leaves, chopped

COOKING STEPS

1. Preheat the air fryer oven to 375°f. Grease pan that will fit inside the air fryer oven.
2. Prepare the frittata crust by mixing the brown rice and flax egg. Press the rice onto the baking dish until you form a crust. Brush with a little oil and cook for 10 minutes.
3. Meanwhile, heat olive oil in a skillet over medium flame and sauté the garlic and onions for 2 minutes.
4. Add the pepper and mushroom and continue stirring for 3 minutes.
5. Stir in the kale, spinach, spring onions, and basil. Remove from the pan and set aside.
6. In a food processor, pulse together the tofu, mustard, turmeric, soy sauce, nutritional yeast, vegan milk and arrowroot powder. Pour in a mixing bowl and stir in the sautéed vegetables.
7. Pour the vegan frittata mixture over the rice crust and cook in the air fryer oven for 40 minutes.

Nutrition: calories 226 fat 05g protein 16g

Coconut curry vegetable rice bowls

5 minutes

40 minutes

Dinner

6 Servings

INGREDIENTS

- 2/3 cup uncooked brown rice
- 1 tsp. Curry powder
- 3/4 tsp. Salt divided
- 1 cup chopped green onion
- 1 cup sliced red bell pepper
- 1 tbsp. Grated ginger
- 1 1/2 tbsp. Sugar
- 1 cup matchstick carrots
- 1 cup chopped red cabbage
- 8 oz. Sliced water chestnuts
- 15 oz. No salt added chickpeas
- 13 oz. Coconut milk

COOKING STEPS

1. Add rice, water, curry powder, and 1/4 tsp. Of the salt in the instant pot. Pressure cook for 15 minutes. Sauté for 2 minutes and serve.

Nutrition: calories 1530 fat 110g carbs 250g protein 80g

Tofu with Sticky Orange Sauce

15 minutes

20 minutes

Dinner

4 Servings

INGREDIENTS

- 1-pound extra-firm tofu drained and pressed (or use super firm tofu)
- 1 teaspoon tamari
- 1 teaspoon cornstarch, (or arrowroot powder)

For sauce:

- 1 teaspoon orange zest
- 1/3 cup oranges juice
- 1/2 cup water
- 2 tablespoons cornstarch (or arrowroot powder)
- 1/4 teaspoon ground pepper flakes
- 1 teaspoon fresh ginger, minced
- 1 tablespoon garlic, minced
- 1 teaspoon pure maple syrup

COOKING STEPS

1   Cut tofu into dices.
2   Put tofu in a Ziploc bag. Add tamarind and seal the bag. Stir the bag until all the tofu is covered with tamarind.
3   Add a tablespoon of cornstarch to the bag. Stir again until the tofu is coated. Set the tofu aside for at least 15 minutes to marinate.
4   Meanwhile, add all the sauce elements to a small bowl and mix with a spoon.
5   Place the tofu in an air fryer. You in all probability want to do this in two batches.
6   Cook the tofu in 390 steps for 10 minutes, adding it for 10 minutes.
7   After you finish cooking the batches of tofu, add it all to a pan on medium-high heat. Give the sauce a stir and pour over the tofu.
8   Mix tofu and sauce until it thickens, and the tofu becomes hot.
9   Serve directly with rice and boiled vegetables if desired.

Nutrition: Calories: 190 Fat: 3g Carbs: 16g Protein: 10g

Green beans and shallots

5 minutes

25 minutes

Side Dish

4 Servings

INGREDIENTS

Preparation time: 5 minutes

Cooking time: 25 minutes

Servings: 4

Ingredients:

- 1½ pounds green beans, trimmed
- Salt and black pepper to taste
- ½ pound shallots, chopped
- ¼ cup walnuts, chopped
- 2 tablespoons olive oil

COOKING STEPS

1. In your air fryer, mix all ingredients and toss.
2. Cook at 350 degrees f for 25 minutes.
3. Divide between plates and serve as a side dish.

Nutrition: calories 182, fat 3, fiber 6, carbs 11, protein 5

Toasty pepper bites

6 minutes   15-30 minutes   Fruit & Vegetables   4 Servings

INGREDIENTS

- 1 medium-sized red bell pepper cut into small pieces
- 1 medium-sized yellow bell pepper cut up into small pieces
- 1 medium-sized green bell pepper cut up into small pieces
- 3 tablespoons of balsamic vinegar
- 2 tablespoon of olive oil
- 1 tablespoon of minced garlic
- 1/2 teaspoon of dried basil
- 1/2 a teaspoon of dried parsley
- Kosher salt as needed
- Pepper as needed

COOKING STEPS

1. Take a mixing bowl and add all of the diced-up bell peppers
2. Mix them well and add olive oil, garlic, balsamic vinegar, basil and parsley
3. Mix them well
4. Season with salt and pepper
5. Stir well
6. Cover and allow it to chill for 30 minutes
7. Preheat your fryer to 390 degrees Fahrenheit
8. Transfer the peppers to your frying basket and cook for 10-15 minutes
9. Serve and enjoy!

Nutrition: Calories: 148 Carbohydrate: 17g Protein: 5g Fat: 7g

Platter of brussels and pine nuts

10 minutes

35 minutes

Fruit & Vegetables

6 Servings

INGREDIENTS

- 15 ounces of brussels sprouts
- 1 tablespoon of olive oil
- 1 and a 3/4 ounce of drained raisins
- Juice of 1 orange
- 1 and a 3/4-ounce toasted pine nuts

COOKING STEPS

1. Take a pot of boiling water and add sprouts, boil for 4 minutes
2. Transfer them to cold water and drain them, store them in a freezer and allow them to cool
3. Take raising and soak them in orange juice for 20 minutes
4. Preheat your fryer to 392 degrees Fahrenheit
5. Take a pan and pour oil and stir fry your sprouts
6. Transfer the sprouts to the cooking basket and roast for 15 minutes
7. Serve the sprouts with a garnish of raisins, pine nuts, orange juice
8. Enjoy!

Nutrition: Calories: 267 Fat: 25g Dietary fiber: 6g Protein: 7g

Vegetable Spring Rolls

10 minutes

35 minutes

Fruit & Vegetables

10 Servings

INGREDIENTS

- 2 cups of cabbage, shredded
- 1 large carrot, cut into thin matchsticks
- 2 large onions, cut into thin matchsticks
- ½ bell pepper, cut into thin matchsticks —any color will work
- 2inch piece ginger, grated
- 8 cloves garlic, minced
- 2 tbsps. of cooking oil plus more for brushing
- a few pinches sugar
- a few pinches salt
- 1 tsp. of soy sauce
- 1 tbsp. of black pepper
- 23 green onions, thinly sliced
- 10 spring roll wrappers
- 2 tbsps. of cornstarch
- water

COOKING STEPS

1. Filling: Get a large bowl then, add the cabbage, carrot, onion, bell pepper, ginger, and garlic.
2. In a medium sauté pan, heat 2 tbsps. oil over high heat adds the filling mixture, stirring in a few pinches of sugar and salt (the sugar helps the vegetables maintain their color).
3. Cook for 23 min, add the soy sauce and black pepper, mix well, and remove from heat. Stir in green onions. Set aside.
4. In a bowl, combine the cornstarch and enough water to make a creamy paste.
5. Fill the rolls: place a tbsp. alternatively, so of filling in the center of each wrapper and roll tightly, dampening the edges with the cornstarch paste to ensure a good seal. Repeat until all the wrappers and filling are used. Alternatively, cut the wrappers into smaller sizes and make mini spring rolls— fun!
6. Briefly, preheat the Air Fryer to 350 degrees F.
7. Brush the rolls with oil, arrange in the Fryer, and cook until crisp and golden, about 20 min, flipping once at the halfway point.

Nutrition: Calories: 154 Fat: 8 g Carbohydrate: 4.3 g Dietary Fiber: 2.4 g

Onion Pakora

5 minutes

20 minutes

Fruit & Vegetables

6 Servings

INGREDIENTS

- 1 cup of graham flour
- ¼ cup of rice flour
- 2 tsps. vegetable oil
- 4 onions, finely chopped
- 2 green chili peppers, finely chopped
- 1 tbsp. of fresh coriander, chopped
- ¼ tsp. of carom
- 1/8 tsp. of chili powder
- turmeric
- salt

COOKING STEPS

1. Put the flours and oil in a bowl. Mix well, adding water as necessary to create a thick, dough like consistency.
2. Add the onions, peppers, coriander, carom, chili powder, and turmeric. Season with salt and mix well.
3. Briefly, preheat the Air Fryer to 350 degrees F.
4. Roll the vegetable mixture into small balls, arrange in the Fryer, and cook until browned, about 6 minutes.
5. Serve with hot sauce and enjoy!

Nutrition: Calories: 119 Fat: 2 g Carbohydrate: 21 g Dietary Fiber: 6 g Protein: 6 g

Vegan Fried Ravioli

10 minutes

10 minutes

Fruit & Vegetables

4 Servings

INGREDIENTS

- ½ cup of panko breadcrumbs
- 1 tsp. of dried oregano
- Pinch salt & pepper
- 2 tsps. of nutritional yeast flakes
- 1 tsp. of dried basil
- 1 tsp. of garlic powder
- ¼ cup of liquid from a can of chickpeas or other beans*
- 8 oz. of frozen or thawed vegan ravioli**
- Spritz cooking spray
- ½ cup of marinara for dipping

COOKING STEPS

1. Mix panko bread. Crumbs, nutritional yeast garlic powder, flakes, dried basil, dried oregano, pepper, and salt.
2. Put aquafaba into a small separate bowl.
3. Dip ravioli into aquafaba and shake off excess liquid then dredge in bread crumb mixture.
4. Put ravioli into the air fryer basket. Proceed until all of the ravioli has been breaded.
5. Sprinkle the ravioli with cooking spray.
6. Set Air Fryer to 390 degrees and air fry for 6 minutes. Flip each ravioli over.
7. Get ravioli from Air Fryer and serve with marinara for dipping.

Nutrition: Calories: 150 Fat: 3g Carbohydrates: 27 g Protein: 5g

Avocado Fries

5 minutes

15 minutes

Fruit & Vegetables

4 Servings

INGREDIENTS

- ½ tsp. of salt
- ½ cup of panko breadcrumbs
- 1 Haas avocado – peeled, pitted, and sliced
- aquafaba from 1 (15 oz.) can white beans or garbanzo beans.

COOKING STEPS

1. In a bowl, toss together the panko and salt. Pour the aquafaba into another bowl.
2. Dredge the avocado slices in the aquafaba in the panko to get a nice, even coating.
3. Arrange the slices in a layer in the Air Fryer basket. A single layer is important.
4. Air Fry for 10 minutes at 390F (without preheating.), shaking after 5 minutes.
5. Serve with your favorite sauce.

To bake:

1. Preheat the oven to 400F. Arrange the slices in a single Air fry for 10 minutes at 390F (without preheating.), shaking after 5 minutes.
2. Lay out on a greased baking sheet. Bake for 20 minutes.
3. Serve with your favorite dipping sauce!

Nutrition: Calories: 711 Fat: 59g Carbohydrates: 21 g Protein: 26g Dietary Fiber: 3.56 g

Crispy Veggie Fries

10 minutes | 10 minutes | Fruit & Vegetables | 3 Servings

INGREDIENTS

- 2 tbsps. of nutritional yeast flakes, divided
- 1 cup of panko breadcrumbs
- Salt and pepper
- 1 cup of rice flour
- 2 tbsps. of Follow Your Heart Vegan Egg powder*
- 2/3 cup of cold water
- Assorted veggies of choice, cut into bitesize chunks or French fry shapes (such as cauliflower, green beans, sweet onions, zucchini or squash)

COOKING STEPS

1. Set up 3 dishes on the counter: Place rice flour in one dish and in another dish whisk the 2/3 cup water, 1 tbsp. of the nutritional yeast flakes and Vegan Egg powder. Whisk until smooth.

2. In the last dish, mix 1 tbsp. of nutritional yeast, the panko breadcrumbs, and pinches of salt and pepper.

3. One veggie fry at a time, dip in the rice flour, followed by Vegan Egg mixture, finally the breadcrumb mixture, pressing gently to set coating. Make as many veggie fries as desired.

4. Lightly spray the Air Fryer basket (or a parchment lined baking sheet. Place the veggie fries in the basket, give them a quick splash of oil and set the fryer at 380degreesF for 8 minutes.

Nutrition: Calories: 134 Fat: 6.6 g Carbohydrates: 13g Protein: 1.5 g Dietary Fiber: 20 g

Air fried carrots, yellow squash & zucchini

 7 minutes   35 minutes   Fruit & Vegetables   4 Servings

INGREDIENTS

- 1 tbsp. Chopped tarragon leaves
- ½tsp. White pepper
- 1 tsp. Salt
- 1pound yellow squash
- 1pound zucchini
- 6 tsp. Olive oil
- ½pound carrots

COOKING STEPS

1. Stem and root the end of squash and zucchini and cut in ¾inch half-moons. Peel and cut carrots into 1inch cubes
2. Combine carrot cubes with 2 tsp. Of olive oil, tossing to combine. Pour into air fryer basket and cook 5 minutes at 400 degrees.
3. As carrots cook, drizzle remaining olive oil over squash and zucchini pieces, then season with pepper and salt. Toss well to coat.
4. Add squash and zucchini when the timer for carrots goes off. Cook 30 minutes, making sure to toss 23 times during the cooking process.
5. Once done, take out veggies and toss with tarragon. Serve up warm!

Nutrition: calories: 122 fat: 9g protein: 6g sugar: 0g

Spaghetti squash tots

 5 minutes 15 minutes Fruit & Vegetables 8-10 Servings

INGREDIENTS

- ¼tsp. Pepper
- ½tsp. Salt
- 1 thinly sliced scallion
- 1 spaghetti squash

COOKING STEPS

1. Wash and cut squash in half lengthwise. Scrape out the seeds.
2. With a fork, remove spaghetti meat by strands and throw out skins.
3. In a clean towel, toss in squash and wring out as much moisture as possible. Place in a bowl and with a knife slice through meat a few times to cut up smaller.
4. Add pepper, salt, and scallions to squash and mix well.
5. Create "tot" shapes with your hands and place in air fryer. Spray with olive oil.
6. Cook 15 minutes at 350 degrees until golden and crispy!

Nutrition: calories: 231 fat: 18g protein: 5g sugar: 0g

Cinnamon butternut squash fries

10 minutes   10 minutes   Fruit & Vegetables   2 Servings

INGREDIENTS

- 1 pinch of salt
- 1 tbsp. Powdered unprocessed sugar
- ½tsp. Nutmeg
- 2 tsp. Cinnamon
- 1 tbsp. Coconut oil
- 10 ounces precut butternut squash fries

COOKING STEPS

1. In a plastic bag, pour in all ingredients. Coat fries with other components till coated and sugar is dissolved.
2. Spread coated fries into a single layer in the air fryer. Cook 10 minutes at 390 degrees until crispy.

Nutrition: calories: 175 fat: 8g protein: 1g sugar: 5g

Cheesy artichokes

 10 minutes
 14 minutes
 Fruit & Vegetables
 4 Servings

INGREDIENTS

- 4 artichokes, trimmed and halved
- 1 cup cheddar cheese, shredded
- 2 tablespoons olive oil
- A pinch of salt and black pepper
- 3 garlic cloves, minced

  1 teaspoon garlic powder

COOKING STEPS

1. In your air fryer's basket, combine the artichokes with the oil, cheese and the other ingredients, toss and cook at 400 degrees f for 14 minutes.
2. Divide everything between plates and serve.

Nutrition: calories 191, fat 8, fiber 2, carbohydrates 12, protein 8

Paprika tomatoes

10 minutes

13 minutes

Fruit & Vegetables

4 Servings

INGREDIENTS

COOKING STEPS

Preparation time: 10 minutes

Cooking time: 15 minutes

Servings: 4

Ingredients:

- 1pound cherry tomatoes, halved
- 1 tablespoon sweet paprika
- 2 tablespoons olive oil
- 2 garlic cloves, minced
- 1 tablespoon lime juice
- 1 tablespoon chives, chopped

1. In your air fryer's basket, combine the tomatoes with the paprika and the other ingredients, toss and cook at a temperature of 370 degrees f for 15 minutes.
2. Divide between plates and serve.

Nutrition: calories 131, fat 4, fiber 7, carbohydrates 10, protein 8

Avocado and tomato salad

 10 minutes   12 minutes   Fruit & Vegetables   4 Servings

INGREDIENTS

- 1pound tomatoes, cut into wedges
- 2 avocados, peeled, pitted and sliced
- 2 tablespoons avocado oil
- 1 red onion, sliced
- 1 tablespoon balsamic vinegar
- Salt and black pepper to the taste
- 1 tablespoon cilantro, chopped

COOKING STEPS

1. In your air fryer, combine the tomatoes with the avocados and the other ingredients, toss and cook at 360 degrees f for 12 minutes.
2. Divide between plates and serve.

Nutrition: calories 144, fat 7, fiber 5, carbohydrates 8, protein 6

Sesame broccoli mix

5 minutes   14 minutes   Fruit & Vegetables   4 Servings

INGREDIENTS

- 1pound broccoli florets
- 1 tablespoon sesame oil
- 1 teaspoon sesame seeds, toasted
- 1 red onion, sliced
- 1 tablespoon lime juice
- 1 teaspoon chili powder
- Salt and black pepper to the taste

COOKING STEPS

1. In your air fryer, combine the broccoli with the oil, sesame seeds and the other ingredients, toss and cook at 380 degrees f for 14 minutes.
2. Divide between plates and serve.

Nutrition: calories 141, fat 3, fiber 4, carbohydrates 4, protein 2

Cabbage sauté

5 minutes   15 minutes   Fruit & Vegetables   4 Servings

INGREDIENTS

- 1pound red cabbage, shredded
- 1 tablespoon balsamic vinegar
- 2 red onions, sliced
- 1 tablespoon olive oil
- 1 tablespoon dill, chopped
- Salt and black pepper to the taste

COOKING STEPS

1. Heat up air fryer with oil at 380 degrees f, add the cabbage, onions and the other ingredients, toss and cook for 15 minutes.
2. Divide between plates and serve.

Nutrition: calories 100, fat 4, fiber 2, carbohydrates 7, protein 2

Tomatoes and kidney beans

10 minutes

20 minutes

Fruit & Vegetables

4 Servings

INGREDIENTS

- 1pound cherry tomatoes, halved
- 1 cup canned kidney beans, drained
- 2 tablespoons balsamic vinegar
- 2 tablespoons olive oil
- 3 garlic cloves, minced
- Salt and black pepper to the taste
- 1 tablespoon chives, chopped

COOKING STEPS

1. In your air fryer, combine the cherry tomatoes with the beans and the other ingredients, toss and cook at 380 degrees f for 20 minutes.
2. Divide between plates and serve.

Nutrition: calories 101, fat 3, fiber 3, carbohydrates 4, protein 2

Glazed mushrooms

 10 minutes   15 minutes   Fruit & Vegetables   4 Servings

INGREDIENTS

- ½ cup low sodium soy sauce
- 4 tablespoons fresh lemon juice
- 1 tablespoon maple syrup
- 4 garlic cloves, finely chopped
- Ground black pepper, as required
- 20 ounces fresh cremini mushrooms, halved

COOKING STEPS

1. Add the soy sauce, lemon juice, maple syrup, garlic and black pepper and mix well. Set aside.
2. Place the mushroom into the greased baking pan in a single layer.
3. Select "air fry" of digital air fryer oven and then adjust the temperature to 350 degrees f.
4. Set the timer for 15 minutes and press "start/stop" to begin cooking.
5. When the unit beeps to show that it is preheated, insert the baking pan in the oven.
6. After 10 minutes of cooking, in the pan, add the soy sauce mixture and stir to combine.
7. When cooking time is complete, remove the mushrooms from oven and serve hot.

Nutrition: calories 70 total fat 3 g total carbohydrates 15 g protein 9 g

Garlic corn

5 minutes

15 minutes

Fruit & Vegetables

4 Servings

INGREDIENTS

- 2cups corn
- 3garlic cloves, minced
- 1tablespoon olive oil
- Juice of 1 lime
- 1teaspoon sweet paprika
- Salt and black pepper to the taste

  2tablespoons dill, chopped

COOKING STEPS

1. Mix the corn with the garlic and the other ingredients in a pan that fits the air fryer, toss, put the pan in the machine and cook at 390 degrees f for 15 minutes.
2. Divide everything between plates and serve.

Nutrition: calories 180, fat 3, fiber 2, carbohydrates 4, protein 6

Lentils and dates brownies with honey and banana flavor

 10 minutes   15 minutes   Dessert   8 Servings

INGREDIENTS

Preparation Time: 10 minutes

Cooking Time: 15 minutes

Servings: 8

Ingredients:

- Canned lentils rinsed and drained 28 ounces.
- Dates 12
- Honey 1 tbsp.
- Banana, peeled and chopped 1
- Baking soda ½ tsp.
- Almond butter 4 tbsp.
- Cocoa powder 2 tbsp.

COOKING STEPS

1. In a container of your food processor, add lentils, butter, banana, cocoa, baking soda, honey and blend it really well.
2. In it then add some dates, some more pulse before pouring it into a greased pan that fits your air fryer and spread evenly. Now bring it to fryer and let it bake for 15 minutes at 360°f.
3. After it's done, take the brownies mix out of the oven and let it cool.
4. Lastly, cut them into pieces before arranging them on a platter to serve.

Nutrition: Calories 162, fat 4, fiber 2, carbs 3, protein 4

Tahini oatmeal chocolate chunk cookies

10 minutes   13 minutes   Dessert   4 Servings

INGREDIENTS

Preparation Time: 10 minutes

Cooking Time: 5 minutes

Servings: 8

Ingredients

- 1/3 cup of tahini
- 1/4 cup of walnuts
- 1/4 cup of maple syrup
- 1/4 cup of Chocolate chunks
- 1/4 tsp of sea salt
- 2 tablespoons of almond flour
- 1 teaspoon of vanilla, it is optional
- 1 cup of gluten free oat flakes

1 teaspoon of cinnamon, it is optional

COOKING STEPS

1. Let the air fryer Preheat to 350 F.
2. In a big bowl, add the maple syrup, cinnamon if used, the tahini, salt, and vanilla if used. Mix well, then add in the walnuts, oat flakes, and almond meal. Then fold the chocolate chips gently.
3. Now the mix is ready, take a full tablespoon of mixture, separate into eight amounts. Wet clean damp hands press them on a baking tray or with a spatula.
4. Place four cookies, or more depending on your air fryer size, line the air fryer basket with parchment paper in one single layer.
5. Let them cook for 5-6 minutes at 350 F, air fry for more minutes if you like them crispy.

Nutrition: calories: 185, fat: 12g, carbohydrates: 15g, protein 12 g

Figs and coconut butter mix

 6 minutes
 4 minutes
 Dessert
 3 Servings

INGREDIENTS

- 2 tablespoons coconut butter
- figs, halved
- ¼ cup sugar
- 1 cup almond, toasted and chopped

COOKING STEPS

1 Put butter in a pan that fits your air fryer and melt over medium high heat.
2 Add figs, sugar and almonds, toss, introduce in your air fryer and cook at 300 degrees f for 4 minutes.
3 Divide into bowls and serve cold.
4 Enjoy!

Nutrition: Calories 170, Fat 4, Fiber 5, Carbs 7, Protein 9

Cocoa and Almonds Bars

30 minutes

4 minutes

Dessert

6 Servings

INGREDIENTS

- ¼ cup cocoa nibs
- 1 cup almonds, drenched and depleted
- 2 tablespoons cocoa powder
- ¼ cup hemp seeds
- ¼ cup goji berries
- ¼ cup coconut, destroyed
  dates, hollowed and drenched

COOKING STEPS

1 Put almonds in your food processor, mix, include hemp seeds, cocoa nibs, cocoa powder, goji, coconut and mix quite well.
2 Add dates, mix well once more, spread on a lined heating sheet that accommodates the air fryer cooker and cook at 320°f for about 4 minutes.
3 Cut into two halves and keep in the cooler for 30 minutes before serving.
4 Enjoy the recipe!

Nutrition: calories 140, fat 6, fiber 3, carbs 7, protein 19

Cashew Bars

INGREDIENTS

Preparation Time: 10 minutes

Cooking Time: 15 minutes

Servings: 6

Ingredients:

- 1/3 cup honey
- ¼ cup almond meal
- 1 tablespoon almond spread
- 1 and ½ cups cashews, hacked
- dates, slashed
- ¾ cup coconut, destroyed
- 1 tablespoon chia seeds

COOKING STEPS

1. In a bowl, blend honey in with almond meal and almond spread and mix well.
2. Add cashews, coconut, dates and chia seeds and mix well once more.
3. Spread this on a lined heating sheet that accommodates the air fryer cooker and press well.
4. Introduce in the fryer and cook at 300°f for about 15 minutes.
5. Leave blend to chill off, cut into medium bars and serve. Enjoy!

Nutrition: calories 121, fat 4, fiber 7, carbs 5, protein 6

Conclusion

Thank you for reading all this book!

If you're looking for the best air fryer, you can't go wrong with a Norpro. This is a great air fryer that is affordable and very easy to use. It has multiple functions and will work in no time.

You have already taken a step towards your improvement.

Best wishes!

CPSIA information can be obtained
at www.ICGtesting.com
Printed in the USA
BVHW090215280421
605947BV00001B/173

9 781802 347845